AF539712

POCKET GUIDE TO
CHEST X-RAYS

2E

This book is dedicated to
Joshua Tamone (1987–2003)
... who will be remembered for his smile ...

PREFACE

In spite of ever-improving sophisticated and advanced medical imaging technology, the chest radiograph remains the most common medical imaging procedure performed. It provides an easily obtained source of information on the heart and lungs—the 'engine room' of the body.

The interpretation of the chest radiograph requires a basic understanding of radiography, a knowledge of chest anatomy and pathology, and a search for radiological clues. This has formed the basis for the chapter layout.

Radiological signs that are seen in computed tomography are included in Appendix 2 because of the overlap with plain film findings and to provide a comprehensive list.

I hope that this pocket guide will provide a good introduction to chest radiology to novice radiologists, chest physicians and cardiothoracic surgeons.

ACKNOWLEDGEMENTS

First edition

Firstly, I am grateful to Anne Streeter for her dedication and helpfulness in typing the complete manuscript from my notes and many changes.

I am thankful to Dr Anne Miller for her contribution of Figures 6.2, 4.2 and 4.11.

I appreciate Professor WSC Hare's permission to reproduce Figure 3.5 from his book *Clinical Radiology for Medical Students and Health Practitioners*.

The publishing team at McGraw-Hill deserve praise for their professionalism and initiation of this project.

Finally, I wish to acknowledge my radiological and clinical colleagues, radiographers, junior medical staff, medical students, nurses and paramedical staff who have stimulated my interest in chest radiology.

Second edition

Once again I am indebted to Anne Streeter for her wonderful secretarial assistance.

I would like to thank Dr Ross Dwyer for his suggested improvements to the first edition. Dr Roger Harris (Chapter 8 'Chest trauma'), Dr Richard Lee (Chapter 9 'Monitoring and support devices') and Dr Kristina Prelog (Chapter 10 'Paediatric overview') also helped to improve the text. I am grateful to Associate Professor Bruno Giuffre for supplying Figures 4.6 and 4.9 and Dr Richard Maher for Figures 4.10, 6.3 and 6.4. GE Australia kindly provided the digital images for Figures 1.3 and 10.1.

GLOSSARY

The glossary is a list of definitions of terms used in chest radiology. Those terms defined in Appendix 2, Signs in Thoracic Radiology, have not been repeated here. The following references give a comprehensive list of recommendations:

- Hansell DM. 'Fleischner Society: Glossary of terms for thoracic imaging'. *Radiology* March 2008; 246(3): 697–722.
- Webb RW, Muller NL, Naidich DP. Illustrated glossary in high-resolution computed tomography terms. In: *High resolution CT of the lung*. 3rd edn. Baltimore: Lippincott Williams & Wilkins, 2001: 599–618.

air bronchogram The bronchus is visible as an air-filled structure surrounded by consolidated or collapsed lung.

airspace The gas-containing part of the lung, including the respiratory bronchioles, but excluding the purely conducting airways.

air-trapping Abnormal retention of air within part of a lung on expiration as a result of airway obstruction.

airway Collective term for air-conducting passages from the larynx to the terminal bronchiole.

architectural distortion Abnormal displacement of lung structures due to lung disease.

atelectasis Collapse and volume loss are synonymous terms.

attenuation (*verb*: attenuate) The process by which the energy of an X-ray beam is reduced as it passes through matter. This reduction is by either absorption or scattering.

bleb A small gas space inside the visceral pleura usually occurring after surgery. Blebs are smaller than bullae and can cause pneumothoraces.

bronchial wall thickening Oedema, inflammatory or neoplastic cells infiltrate the peribronchial interstitial space.

bronchiectasis Bronchial dilatation which often has associated bronchial wall thickening.

bulla (*plural*: bullae; *adjective*: bullous) An emphysematous space which normally has a very thin wall and communicates with the bronchial tree. The bulla is more than 1 cm in size and, if ruptured, can cause a pneumothorax.

calcification (*adjective*: calcified) Deposition of calcium salts within a structure rendering it visible on X-ray examination.

cavity Thick-walled space containing air, or air and fluid with an air–fluid level.

consolidation Filling of the airspaces with abnormal material, such as transudate, exudate, cells or protein. Consolidated lung characteristically appears dense and shows the bronchi as air-filled tubular structures (see air bronchogram sign, Appendix 2) but obscures the underlying vessels.

cor pulmonale In the presence of severe lung disease the right heart becomes dilated. The central pulmonary arteries become dilated because of the pulmonary hypertension.

cyst Thin-walled space containing either air or fluid.

density General non-specific term for any area of whiteness on the chest radiograph.

end-stage lung This is the final common appearance of a number of chronic infiltrative lung diseases and is characterised by the presence of fibrosis, alveolar loss, bronchiolectasis and disruption of normal lung architecture.

flail chest A chest wall injury that disturbs the mechanics of ventilation because of the abnormal mobility. It occurs when there are more than five contiguous single fractures or when there are three or more double rib fractures. Typically associated with lung injury and possibly extrathoracic injury.

ground-glass opacity Hazy increase in lung density which is less than consolidation and still allows visualisation of the vessels.

hilum (*plural*: hila; *adjective*: hilar; *old term*: hilus) The hilum is an imprecisely defined anatomical region which is the junction area between the mediastinum and lung.

interstitium (*adjective*: interstitial) The loose connective tissue that forms the structure for the lungs. It includes the connective tissues around the bronchi and vessels and the interlobular septae. It is not normally visible radiographically but thickens with disease processes.

kVp The peak kilovoltage across an X-ray tube. A higher kVp produces higher energy X-rays.

lucency (*adjective*: lucent) An area of blackness on the radiograph due to the transmission of X-rays through matter. (*synonyms*: translucency, transradiancy)

mA (milliampere/second) The amount of current through an X-ray tube. It determines the quantity of the X-rays generated to produce an image.

mass A discrete opacity > 3 cm in size.

mycetoma Fungus ball.

nodule A discrete opacity < 3 cm in size.

nosocomial pneumonia A general term for hospital-acquired pneumonia.

opacity Synonym for density.

pneumatocoele Thin-walled, transient, gas-filled space in the lungs; seen with staphylococcal and *Pneumocystis jirovecii* pneumonia; also seen after trauma and hydrocarbon pneumonia. It is presumed that it is a tension cyst due to obstruction of a bronchiole.

pneumomediastinum Air present in the mediastinum outside the oesophagus and tracheobronchial tree.

pneumopericardium Air present in the pericardial space.

pneumothorax Free gas in the pleural space (i.e. between the parietal and visceral pleura). It may be modified by the prefixes hydro-, pyo-, haemo- and chylo-.

reticular shadowing Fine, medium or coarse irregular linear opacities due to interstitial thickening.

tomogram A special radiograph in which one plane is in focus with the planes above and below blurred out. It is achieved by moving the X-ray tube and cassette in different directions during exposure.

Valsalva manoeuvre Forced expiration against a closed glottis. This produces an increase in thoracic pressure.

COMMON ABBREVIATIONS AND ACRONYMS

ABMA	antibasement membrane antibody
ABPA	allergic bronchopulmonary aspergillosis
AI	aortic insufficiency
AIDS	acquired immunodeficiency syndrome
AILD	angioimmunoblastic lymphadenopathy
AIP	acute interstitial pneumonia
ALI	acute lung injury
AMBER	advanced multiple beam equalisation radiography
AMI	acute myocardial infarction
ANCA	antineutrophil cytoplasmic antibodies
AP	anteroposterior
APO	acute pulmonary oedema
ARDS	adult respiratory distress syndrome
AS	aortic stenosis
ASD	atrial septal defect
AVF	arteriovenous fistula
BAC	bronchioalveolar carcinoma
BAL	bronchoalveolar lavage
BALT	bronchus-associated lymphoma tumour (see MALT)
BCG	bacille Calmette-Guérin
BHL	bilateral hilar lymphadenopathy
BIP	bronchiolitis obliterans and diffuse interstitial pneumonia
BOOP	bronchiolitis obliterans with organising pneumonia
CABG	coronary artery bypass graft
CAD	computer-aided diagnosis
CAD	coronary artery disease
CAL	chronic airways limitation
CAT	computerised axial tomography
CCF	congestive cardiac failure
CD4	a type of T lymphocyte using the cluster of differentiation (CD) classification

CDS	ciliary dyskinesia syndrome
CECT	contrast-enhanced computed tomography
CF	cystic fibrosis
CFA	crytogenic fibrosing alveolitis
CID	cytomegalic inclusion disease
CIP	chronic interstitial pneumonitis
CLL	chronic lymphocytic leukemia
CMV	cytomegalovirus
COAD	chronic obstructive airways disease
COP	cryptogenic organising pneumonia
COPD	chronic obstructive pulmonary disease
CPFE	combined pulmonary fibrosis and emphysema
CREST	calcinosis, Raynaud syndrome, oesophageal dysmotility, sclerodactyly and telangiectasia
CRT	cardiac resynchronisation therapy
CRT-D	defibrillator
CSF	cerebral spinal fluid
CT	computed tomography
CTEPH	chronic thromboembolic pulmonary hypertension
CTPA	computed tomographic pulmonary angiography
CTR	cardiothoracic ratio
CWP	coal workers' pneumoconiosis
CXR	chest X-ray (chest radiograph)
DAD	diffuse alveolar damage
DCS	dyskinetic cilia syndrome
DD	differential diagnosis
DIC	disseminated intravascular coagulation
DIP	desquamative interstitial pneumonia
DPH	diffuse pulmonary haemorrhage
DR	digital radiography
DVT	deep venous/vein thrombosis
EAA	extrinsic allergic alveolitis
ECG	electrocardiogram
ECMO	extracorporeal membrane oxygenation
EG	eosinophilic granuloma
ESL	end-stage lung
ETT	endotracheal tube
GBM	glomerular basement membrane
GGO	ground-glass opacity
GIP	giant cell interstitial pneumonia
HIV	human immunodeficiency virus
HMD	hyaline membrane disease
HPOA	hypertrophic pulmonary osteoarthropathy

HP	hypersensitivity pneumonia
HRCT	high-resolution computed tomography
HU	Hounsfield units
IACPB	intra-aortic counterpulsation balloon also known as 'aortic balloon pump'
ICC	intercostal catheter
II	image intensifier
ILD	interstitial lung disease
INH	isonicotinic acid hydrazide (isoniazid)
IPF	idiopathic pulmonary fibrosis
IPH	idiopathic pulmonary haemosiderosis
IVC	inferior vena cava
LAM	lymphangioleiomyomatosis
LDH	lactate dehydrogenase
LIP	lymphocytic interstitial pneumonia
LVRS	lung volume reduction surgery
MAC	*Mycobacterium avium-intracellulare* complex
MAI	*Mycobacterium avium-intracellulare*
MALT	mucosa-associated lymphoid tissue
MI	mitral incompetence
MOT	*Mycobacterium* other than tuberculosis
MRI	magnetic resonance imaging
MS	mitral stenosis
NAI	non-accidental injury
NF	neurofibromatosis
NSIP	non-specific interstitial pneumonia
NTM	non-tuberculous *Mycobacterium*
OSA	obstructive sleep apnoea
PA	posteroanterior
PACS	picture archiving and communication system
PAH	pulmonary arterial hypertension
PAOP	pulmonary artery occlusion pressure
PAP	pulmonary alveolar proteinosis
PAPVR	partial anomalous pulmonary venous return
PAWP	pulmonary artery wedge pressures
PCP	*Pneumocystis jirovecii* (*carinii*) pneumonia
PCWP	pulmonary capillary wedge pressure
PDA	patent ductus arteriosus
PE	pulmonary embolism
PEEP	positive end-expiratory pressure
PET	positron emission tomography
PICC	peripherally inserted central catheter
PIE (adult)	pulmonary infiltrate with eosinophilia

PIE (neonate)	pulmonary interstitial emphysema
PIOPED	prospective investigation of pulmonary embolism diagnosis study
PLCH	pulmonary Langerhans cell histiocytosis
PMF	progressive massive fibrosis
PNET	primitive neuroectodermal tumour
PPD	purified protein derivative of tuberculin
PPV	positive pressure ventilation
PTLD	post-transplant lymphoproliferative disorder
RB	respiratory bronchiolitis, as in RB-ILD
RML	right middle lobe
RMLS	right middle lobe syndrome
RSV	respiratory syncytial virus
SARS	severe acute respiratory syndrome
SCUBA	self-contained underwater breathing apparatus
SIADH	syndrome of inappropriate secretion of antidiuretic hormone
SLE	systemic lupus erythematosus
SOBOE	shortness of breath on exertion
SPN	solitary pulmonary nodule
SVC	superior vena cava
TAPVR	total anomalous pulmonary venous return
TB	tuberculosis
TIPS	transjugular intrahepatic portosystemic shunt
TNM	tumour–node–metastasis staging system
TOE	transoesophageal echocardiography
TOF	tracheo-oesophageal fistula
TPN	total parenteral nutrition
TRALI	transfusion related acute lung injury
TS	tuberous sclerosis
UIP	usual interstitial pneumonia
URTI	upper respiratory tract infection
US	ultrasound
VATER	vertebral/vascular, anal, cardiac, tracheo-oesophageal, renal/radial anomalies
VATS	video-assisted thorascopic surgery
VILI	ventilator-induced lung injury
V/Q	ventilation/perfusion isotope scan
VSD	ventricular septal defect

CHAPTER 1

INTRODUCTION TO TECHNIQUES

CHEST RADIOGRAPH

X-rays were discovered in 1895 by Conrad Roentgen, a German physicist. They are a form of energy and are part of the electromagnetic spectrum, lying between gamma rays and ultraviolet light. They are produced when a stream of electrons in a vacuum tube passes from the cathode and strikes the anode. Because of their short wavelength, X-rays can penetrate materials that do not transmit visible light. However, different degrees of absorption and penetration of the X-rays occur as they pass in a straight line through the body because of the varying tissue densities. The X-rays exiting from the body can expose photosensitive film to allow us to record these different densities within the body. For example, very little absorption occurs in the lungs and the X-rays pass through to expose the film black, whereas the bones absorb the X-rays and, with reduced exposure, the film is white. If the lung airspaces become filled in disease processes, the denser or consolidated lungs appear whiter on the radiograph.

The plain chest radiograph, colloquially called the chest X-ray (CXR), is the most commonly performed imaging procedure in most radiology practices. The standard frontal chest radiograph is with the beam of X-rays in a posteroanterior (PA) direction relative to the patient. The front of the patient is against the film cassette with the X-ray tube about 2–4 m behind. The radiographer centres the beam on the T4 vertebra and instructs patients to put their wrists on their hips to displace the scapulae laterally so as not to obscure the lung fields.

Conventional chest radiography (60–80 kVp) has been improved using higher energy X-rays produced with a higher kilovoltage. With a high kilovoltage technique (120–140 kVp), the bony structures appear less dense and permit better visualisation of the mediastinum and more of the lung parenchyma. The only disadvantage is the reduced visualisation of calcific densities in the lungs. A grid or air gap is used to reduce scatter radiation exposing the film.

The ideal studies are the PA erect and left lateral view radiographs obtained on full inspiration, so that maximal lung volume is visualised.

Many ill patients need to be radiographed in bed with anteroposterior (AP) projections. These views produce reduced diagnostic information but fortunately are only needed to exclude or confirm major disease processes or are only performed to evaluate line or tube placement (see Fig. 1.1).

Fig. 1.1 (a) Posteroanterior (PA) versus (b) anteroposterior (AP) views of the chest

Wherever possible the frontal film should ideally be a PA study. Even in the X-ray department, the patient may be unable to stand for a PA view so an AP view is performed. Not all AP views are the same technique and therefore are of varying quality. They could be departmental or 'mobile', erect or supine.

The AP mobile film should be used for ill patients who have difficulty moving and where space is limited at the bedside. Because of the longer exposure times required for an AP film and the expected poorer centring, the film quality is not as good. Fortunately, the AP film is good for showing lines and catheters and gross pleural and pulmonary disease but magnification spoils assessment of cardiac size. The supine AP film is restricted to very ill patients or those patients who cannot sit up. The AP supine film will be less helpful than the AP erect film in showing pleural effusions.

It is mandatory for the radiograph to be labelled 'AP' by the radiographer. If such labelling is missing, clues include the position of the scapulae, shape of the ribs and the smaller visible lung volumes.

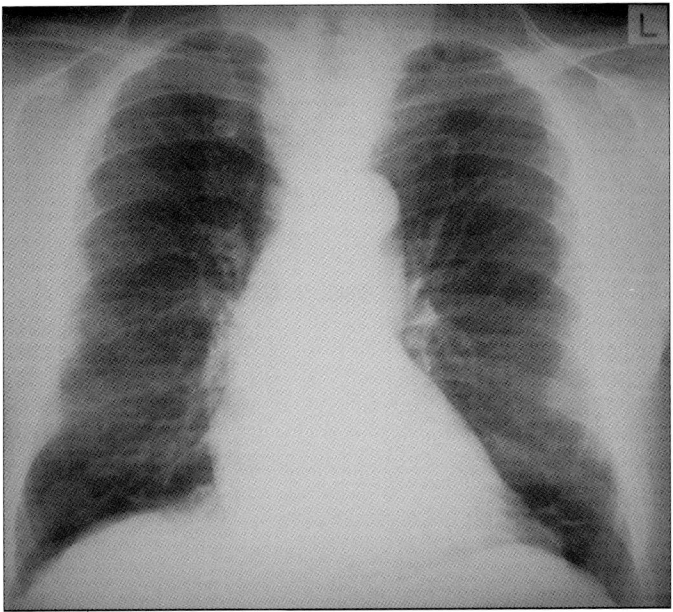

FIG 1.1a

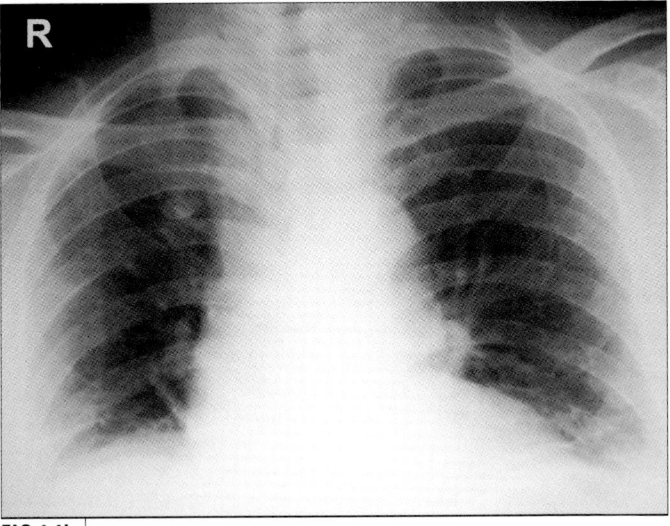

FIG 1.1b

TABLE 1.1 Radiographic views

Projections/techniques	Indication
PA	Varied
AP (department or mobile) (erect or supine)	Ill patient
Expiration	Pneumothorax, air-trapping
Oblique	Rib fracture, pleural plaques
Lordotic	Apical and middle lobe disease
Lateral decubitus	Pleural effusion, pneumothorax
Lateral shoot-through	Pneumothorax

Other projections include supine expiratory, oblique, lordotic, reverse lordotic, penetrated or lateral decubitus views (see Table 1.1 and Fig. 1.2).

The X-ray film is protected within a cassette, which also contains intensification screens. The intensification screens produce light to augment the X-ray exposure of the photosensitive film and allow a reduction in the amount of irradiation required for the patient. Recent improvements are faster film emulsions, faster intensification screens, wide-latitude film and asymmetric film–screen combinations.

The technical challenge in chest radiography is the big contrast difference between the lungs (air density), mediastinum (soft tissue density) and the bones (calcific density). The mediastinum attenuates (absorbs) the X-rays about ten times more than the lungs.

Recent technical improvements are digital systems that use selenium-based, flat-panel detectors or storage phosphor systems with either hard-copy (film) or soft-copy viewing on a *cathode ray tube* (CRT) monitor. The monitors with a 2000 × 2000 matrix (pixel size, 0.2 mm) are better.

Digital radiography produces a digital image, which is simply a representation of a picture as a two-dimensional array of numbers. Each number represents a single picture element (pixel) in the image. The value of each pixel defines the brightness, or greyscale value, of that point in the image. Dual energy radiography is an imaging technique where a low kVp image and high kVp are acquired in rapid succession. The acquired images are computer processed to create a soft tissue image for the lungs and a bone image, in addition to the standard image. These dual energy subtraction views improve the conspicuity of lung and bone pathology (see Fig. 1.3) A new advance

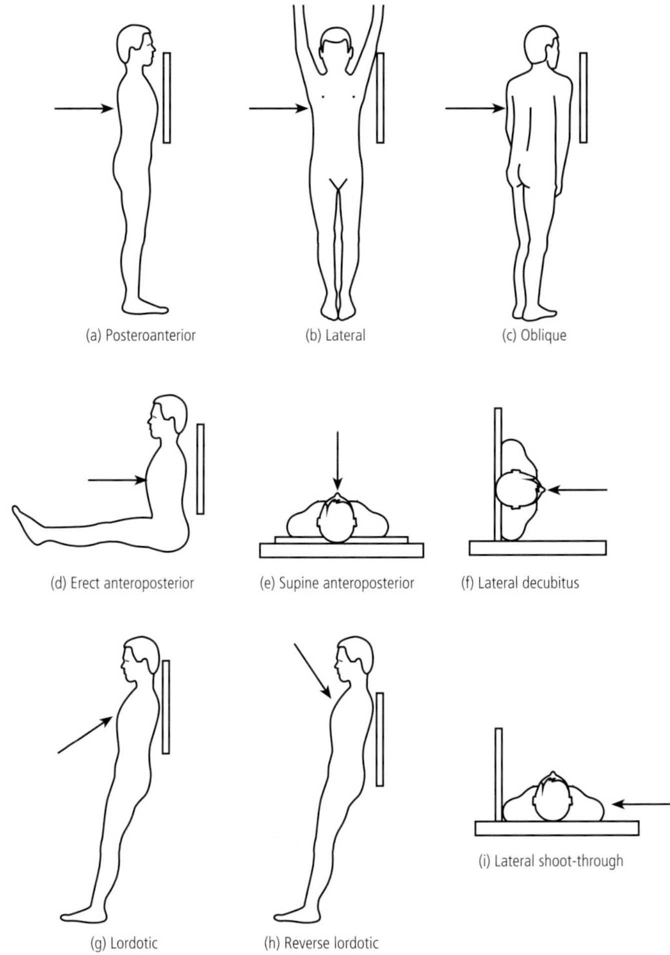

Fig. 1.2 Chest radiographic projections

is 'computer aided diagnosis', where abnormal areas are highlighted for the radiologist's attention.

The digital systems have advantages in image acquisition, transmission, display and storage. The digital data can be used in *picture archiving and communication systems* (PACS), that is, the retrieval and transmission of the image over telephone lines.

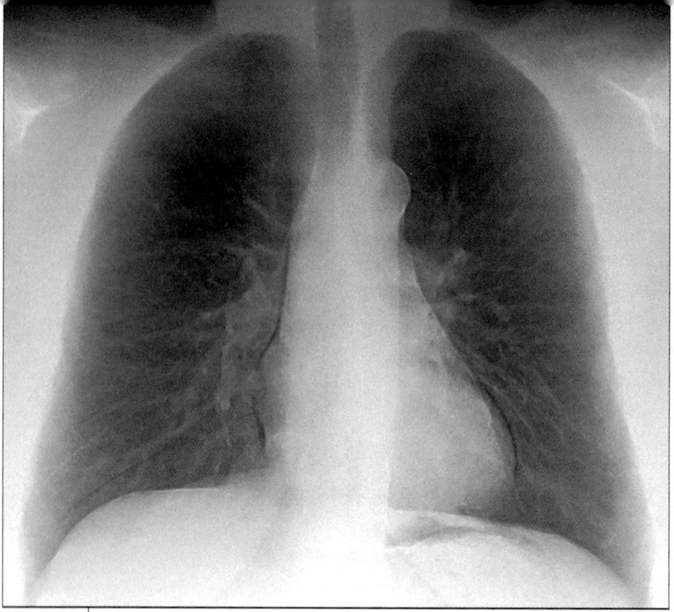

FIG 1.3a

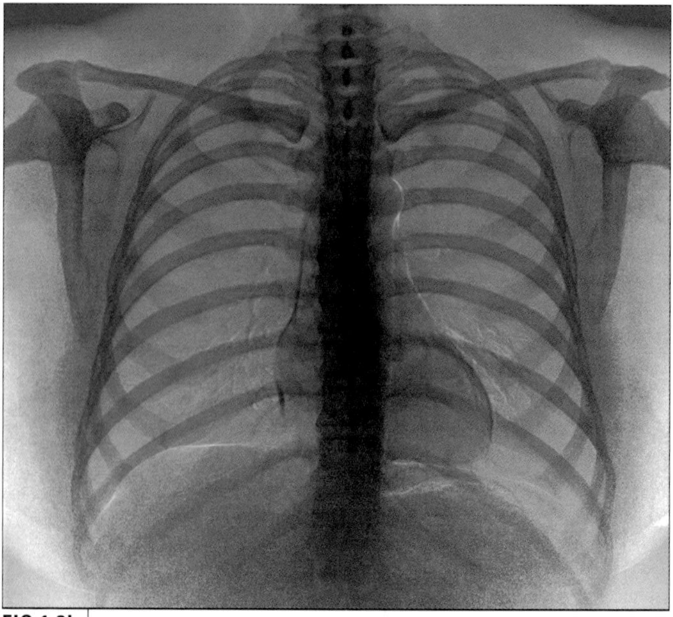

FIG 1.3b

Fig. 1.3 Dual energy subtractions

(a) Lung and soft tissue view. The bones have been subtracted and the lung detail is superb. **(b)** Bone view. The lungs and soft tissue have been subtracted with the bones perfectly visualised.

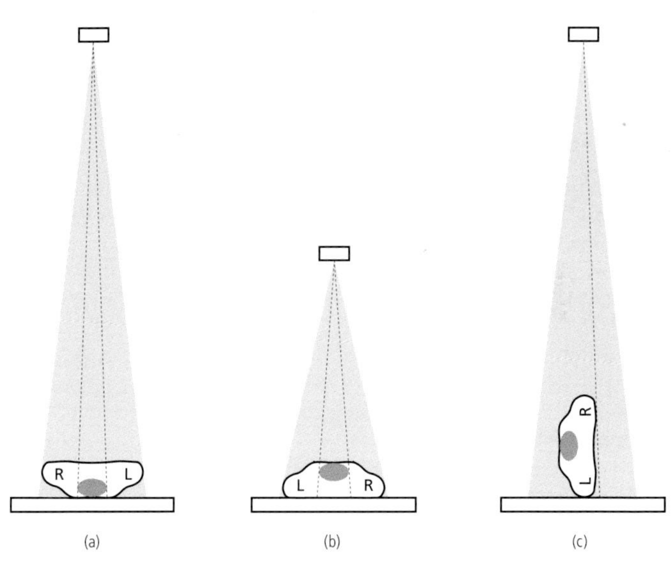

Fig. 1.4 Standard projections

(a) PA radiograph reflects the true size of the heart; **(b)** AP radiograph shows the heart larger because of beam diversion; **(c)** left lateral radiograph magnifies the right ribs and projects them behind the left ribs.

Radiation dose

In modern chest radiography during a routine PA exposure, the lungs receive about 150 μGy (15 millirad) of radiation, the gonads about 10 μGy (1 millirad) and the skin entry dose is 500 μGy (50 millirad). The probability of a fatal cancer being induced in an individual patient from a single frontal radiograph is estimated at one per million.

In computed tomography (CT) the dose is higher by a factor of 100 and is equivalent to the background radiation that people are exposed to each year.

FLUOROSCOPY

Fluoroscopy is the process of viewing on a monitor a real-time image produced by a continuous, low power X-ray beam. The X-ray beam passes through the body and stimulates an image intensifier (II), which converts the signal into a television image. This method is used to screen the diaphragmatic movements and to aid arteriography and interventional procedures, such as lung tumour biopsy.

Fluoroscopy can be used for uncooperative children to check for possible air trapping due to a bronchial foreign body.

A cinetracheogram, either with fluoroscopy or CT scanning, can show the dynamic collapse of the trachea and main bronchi with coughing in tracheomalacia.

COMPUTED TOMOGRAPHY

CT is a non-invasive diagnostic technique that provides more information than the standard radiograph but uses more radiation. The images are more sensitive in detecting abnormalities and provide better anatomic detail.

A narrow, collimated beam of revolving X-rays is transmitted through the body to a ring of detectors to give a cross-sectional image. The density of small volumes (voxels) in the body can be calculated with computers from the multiple projections. The CT image itself is composed of a matrix of picture elements (pixels).

The density of each voxel is measured in Hounsfield units (HU). The reference value for water is 0 HU and for air is –1000 HU.

In spiral/helical scanning, the patient is moved through the CT gantry on the sliding table top at a constant rate while being scanned. The variable factors are the speed of travel, slice thickness and scan length. The ratio of the table movement occurring during a complete tube rotation to the slice thickness is referred to as the 'pitch'. The data can be rapidly acquired on a single breath hold. Multidetector scanners allow even faster data acquisition, greater anatomic coverage, optimal contrast enhancement and improved spatial resolution.

High-resolution CT (HRCT) scanning shows fine detail of the lung by using thin sections (1 mm) and a high-frequency spatial reconstruction algorithm.

MAGNETIC RESONANCE IMAGING (MRI)

MRI is a non-invasive diagnostic technique that uses external magnetic fields and radiofrequency waves to produce an image. When the patient lies in an MRI scanner, the hydrogen nuclei in water and fat molecules within the body become aligned with the magnetic field. When a special pulse of radiofrequency energy is applied, the nuclei are initially flipped but then return to their original state. The change in energy level and spin, which are different for various tissues, are measured and converted by computers into a greyscale image.

In the thorax, the main uses are for assessment of apical lung tumours, aortic dissection and cardiac motion. Inhaled hyperpolarised helium-3 can be used to study regional lung ventilation (as with isotope scanning).

ISOTOPE SCANNING

Isotope scanning uses various radioactive labelled agents to detect abnormalities. The main nuclear medicine studies in the thorax are:

- ventilation and perfusion scanning (V/Q scan), using radioactive gas and technetium-99 albumin microspheres to detect pulmonary emboli
- myocardial infarct imaging with thallium-201
- technetium-labelled phosphonates for bony secondary deposits
- positron emission tomography (PET)—the uptake of the radiopharmaceutical fluoro-2-deoxy-d-glucose (FDG) is used to help stage lung carcinoma. Most PET scanners are combined with multislice CT scanners to improve spatial resolution.

ULTRASOUND

Ultrasound is sound waves with a frequency above the human hearing range. Ultrasound waves are produced by a piezoelectric crystal in the transducer probe, which also detects their returning signal. The echo signal is converted into an electrical signal and this is subsequently processed into a greyscale picture.

Ultrasound is helpful in localising pleural effusions to facilitate drainage. Doppler ultrasound can be used to assess blood flow velocities and is a non-invasive technique of diagnosing deep vein thrombosis.

PULMONARY ANGIOGRAPHY

In pulmonary angiography, a catheter is passed via a peripheral vein, usually the right common femoral vein, through the right side of the heart to selectively catheterise the pulmonary artery. The injected contrast shows the pulmonary arterial and venous circulations. Pulmonary angiography is the previously flawed 'gold standard' for detection of pulmonary emboli. CT pulmonary angiography is the new gold standard, although it too is not perfect.

BRONCHIAL ANGIOGRAPHY

Selective catheterisation of the bronchial arteries may be required to demonstrate the site and cause of haemoptysis. This study is needed before bronchial artery embolisation.

INTERVENTIONAL PROCEDURES

- Lung biopsy. Under fluoroscopic or CT guidance, a needle can be inserted into a pulmonary, pleural or mediastinal mass. The aspirated material is used for cytological and microbiological analysis.
- Abscess and empyema drainage. A catheter can be introduced percutaneously under imaging guidance to drain pus collections.
- Pleural fluid aspiration. A needle can be inserted into small effusions under ultrasound guidance and a specimen aspirated for analysis.
- Bronchial artery embolisation. Embolic material, such as coils (cotton-coated metallic threads), can be used to occlude bleeding bronchial arteries caused by bronchiectasis.

CHAPTER 2

BASIC RADIOLOGIC ANATOMY

A basic knowledge of chest anatomy is needed to understand the appearances on the chest X-ray (CXR). In CXR interpretation, the first decision is whether the appearances are normal or not. Only with a sound knowledge of the radiologic anatomy can the interpretation proceed. With experience, the radiologist becomes aware of differences in anatomy due to body habitus, degree of inspiration and position of the patient.

CHEST ANATOMY

Airways

The normal adult trachea is 1.5–1.8 cm wide, midline in the lower neck and deviates slightly to the right as it lies on the right side of the aortic arch. In cadaveric anatomy and on expiration, the carina lies at the T4 level. On inspiration the carina will move inferiorly to the T6 level. In adults, the right main bronchus has a steeper angle than does the left but the angles are symmetrical in children.

The adult right main bronchus is 2.5 cm long and is 25° from the vertical, whereas the left main bronchus is 4.5 cm long and 45° from the vertical. The difference is due to the early origin of the right upper lobe bronchus (see Fig. 2.1). The intermediate bronchus continues for 2.5 cm before dividing into the middle and right lower lobe bronchi.

The more vertical orientation of the right main bronchus explains why an over-advanced endotracheal tube enters it and can obstruct the right upper lobe bronchus or left lung (see Fig. 2.2).

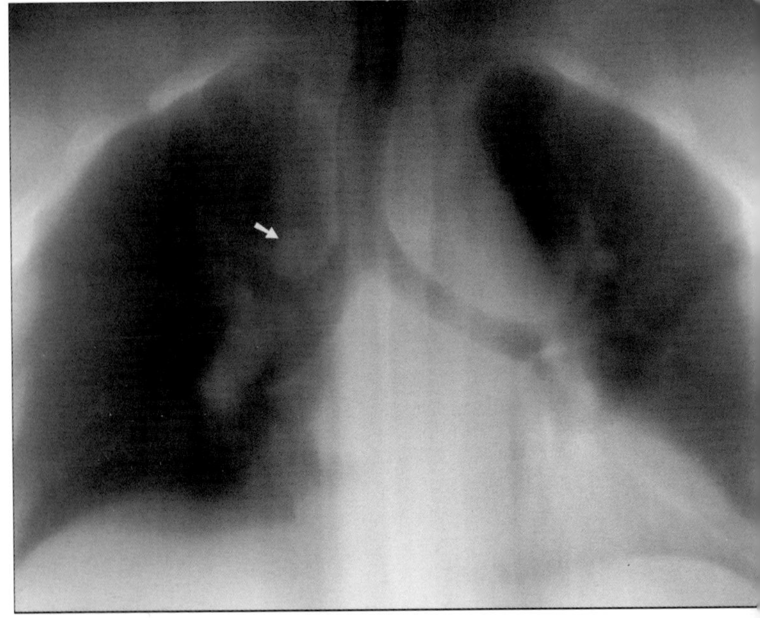

Fig. 2.1 Tracheal tomogram
The conventional tomogram has been produced by movement of the X-ray tube and film so that only the plane in focus is not blurred. In this case, the anatomy of the trachea and main bronchi is well seen. Note the azygous vein, prominent with patient supine, at the right tracheobronchial angle coming forward to drain into the superior vena cava (SVC).

The right upper lobe bronchus originates above the level of the pulmonary artery and is called by some authors the 'eparterial bronchus'. All the other lobar arteries arise below the pulmonary artery and are 'hyparterial'.

The lobar bronchi divide into segmental bronchi to supply the corresponding lung segments (see Table 2.1 on page 16).

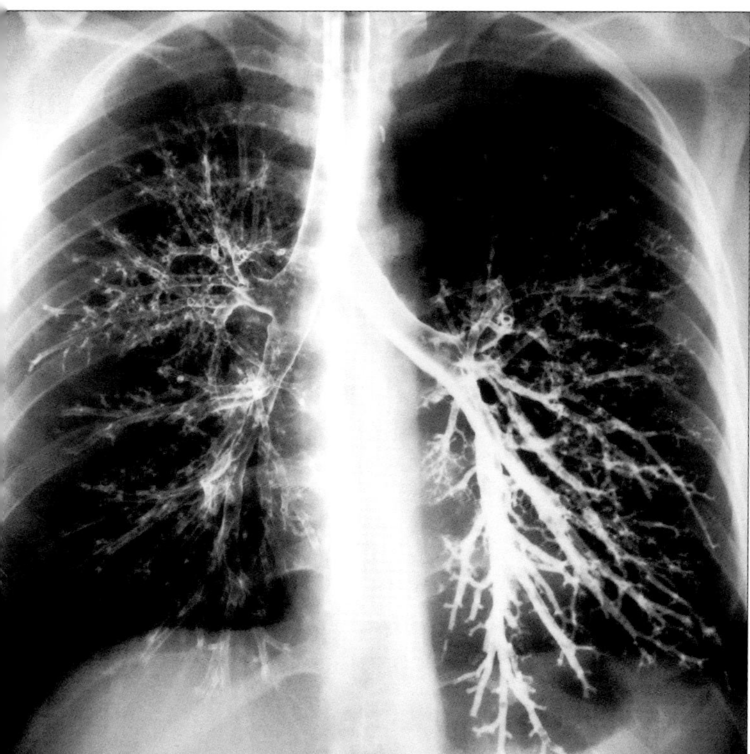

Fig 2.2 Bronchial anatomy

Brochiograms are an outmoded imaging technique where special iodine-based contrast media were instilled into the bronchial tree. With tipping and gravity, all the segmental bronchi were able to be outlined. These studies were useful to demonstrate bronchiectasis. Note the asymmetry in the right and left bronchi with the right upper lobe bronchus arising early.

Lungs

Each lung is divided into lobes by the interlobar fissures, which are reflections of the visceral pleura: the right lung has three lobes—upper, middle and lower; the left lung has two lobes—upper and lower. The lungs are further subdivided into ten segments on the right and eight segments on the left. On the left side, the equivalent of the middle lobe is the lingular segments of the upper lobe (see Fig. 2.3, overleaf, and Table 2.1 on page 16).

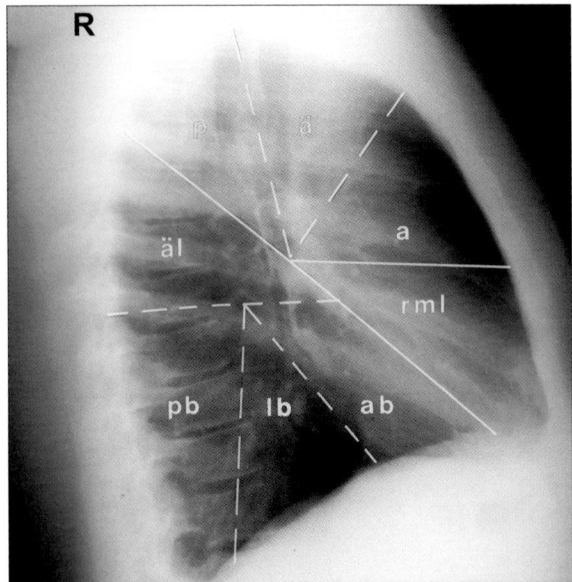

FIG 2.3a

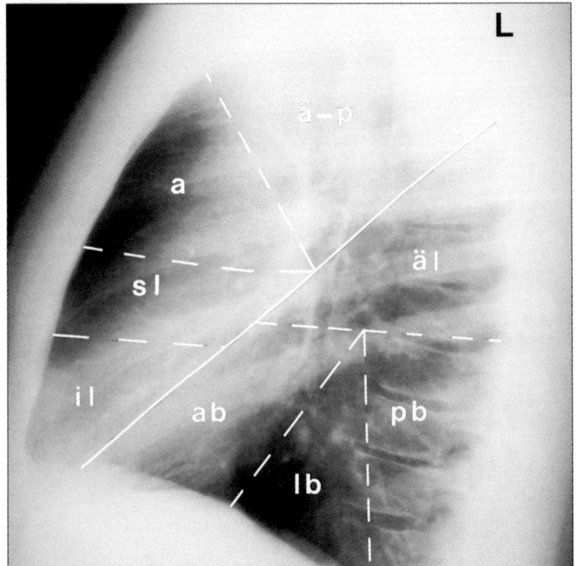

FIG 2.3b

Fig. 2.3 Segmental bronchi and lung segments (a) right lateral view; (b) left lateral view; (c) PA view

The lung segments fit together in the lung like a three-dimensional jigsaw. They correspond to the bronchial divisions. There are ten segments in the right lung and eight segments in the left. The numbering system is shown in Table 2.1, overleaf. For example, the bronchus in the apical segment of the lower lobe is called B6. The lingular segments of the left upper lobe correspond to the middle lobe; there is no left medial basal segment as this space is occupied by the heart; the apical and posterior segments of the left upper lobe are fused. Note that the interlobar (oblique) fissures pass from about 4 cm behind the anterior costophrenic angle through the hilum to T4.

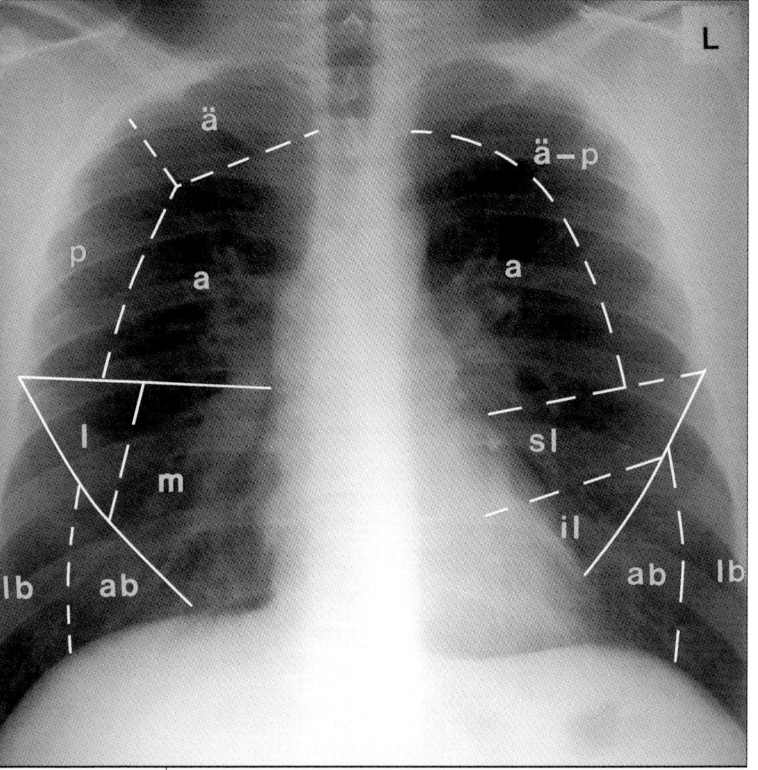

FIG 2.3c

TABLE 2.1 Segmental bronchi and lung segments

Right upper lobe			**Left upper lobe**		
B1	ä	apical	B1, B3	ä-p	apicoposterior
B2	a	anterior	B2	a	anterior
B3	p	posterior			
Right middle lobe					
B4	l	lateral	B4	sl	superior lingula
B5	m	medial	B5	il	inferior lingula
Right lower lobe			**Left lower lobe**		
B6	äl	apical lower	B6	äl	apical lower
B7	mb	medial basal			
B8	ab	anterior basal	B7, B8	ab	anteromedial basal
B9	lb	lateral basal	B9	lb	lateral basal
B10	pb	posterior basal	B10	pb	posterior basal

The fissures are incomplete in the majority of patients but are important landmarks in lobar anatomy. However, the fissures are an inconstant finding, with the horizontal fissure only seen in 50% of chest radiographs.

The major interlobar (oblique) fissure on each side passes obliquely as a plane from '4 to 4', that is, from 4 cm behind the anterior costophrenic angle through the hilum to the T4 level (as seen on the lateral view). In the right lung, the major fissure separates the lower lobe from the upper and middle lobes; in the left lung, it separates the upper and lower lobes. The horizontal fissure (or minor fissure) separates the middle lobe from the upper lobe. It lies at the level of the fourth costal cartilage and contacts the lateral chest wall near the axillary portion of the right sixth rib.

An accessory fissure separates a lung segment or part of a lobe from the remainder of a lobe. The commonest accessory fissure is the azygos fissure, present in about 0.5% of the population. The azygos lobe is formed when the azygos vein invaginates the right upper lobe during gestation creating a portion of lung between the azygos fissure and the mediastinum. The azygos fissure consists of four layers of pleura (two parietal and two visceral) and contains the arch of the azygos vein inferiorly. On the frontal film, the azygos fissure has an inverted comma shape with the azygos vein having a teardrop appearance at the inferior extent of the fissure.

For convenience, the lung fields can be divided into upper, mid and lower zones. The upper zones lie above the level of the second costal cartilage; the mid-zones between the levels of the second and fourth costal cartilages; and the lower zones below the level of the fourth costal cartilage. The apices lie above the clavicles.

Lung parenchyma

The bronchial tree continues dividing into smaller and smaller bronchi until they lose their cartilage and become bronchioles. The terminal bronchiole is the last exclusively conducting structure. Beyond the terminal bronchioles lie the respiratory bronchioles, the alveolar ducts, alveolar sacs and alveoli—the gas-exchanging units of the lung.

The *acinus* is that portion of the lung distal to the terminal bronchiole, comprising the respiratory bronchioles, alveolar ducts, alveolar sacs and alveoli; it is about 5 mm in diameter.

Several acini are grouped together into a *secondary pulmonary lobule*, which is about 2 cm in diameter and polyhedral in shape. The secondary pulmonary lobules are separated from each other by connective tissue (interlobular septa). The secondary pulmonary lobule is, therefore, the smallest discrete portion of lung surrounded by connective tissue septa. The interlobular septa contain the lymphatics and venules. Thickening of the septa is seen as Kerley B lines.

In the centre of each secondary pulmonary lobule are the bronchovascular bundles, which are made up of the preterminal bronchiole and its accompanying artery.

The primary pulmonary lobule of Miller consists of all the alveolar ducts, alveolar sacs and alveoli distal to the last respiratory bronchiole. This unit is of no practical radiographic significance.

Besides the airspaces and vessels, an important morphological component of the parenchyma is the interstitium (see Fig. 2.4). The interstitial compartment is the supportive framework of the lung. At a microscopic level, the interstitial connective tissue is composed of cells, collagen and elastic fibres. The axial interstitium extends out from the hilum supporting the bronchovascular bundles and continuing into each secondary pulmonary lobule around the centrilobular artery and bronchus.

The peripheral interstitium extends from the subpleural interstitium, beneath the visceral pleura, into the lung as the interlobular septa. The interlobular septa contain the lymphatics and venules. Thickening of the interlobular septa is seen as Kerley B lines.

Pulmonary vessels

The pulmonary arteries extend in a tree-like manner from the hilum to the lungs (see Fig. 2.5). These branching, blood-filled band opacities (lung markings) are well seen against the air-filled lung. The veins drain back to the left atrium. In the upper lobes the vessels have a vertical orientation with the veins lateral to the arteries. In the lower

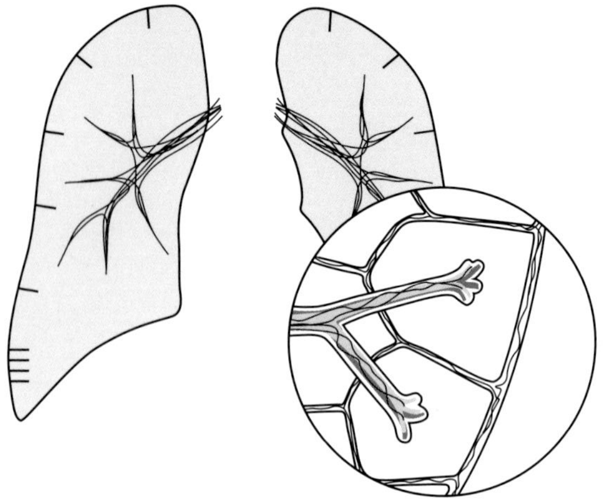

Fig. 2.4 The pulmonary interstitium
The axial and peripheral interstitium provide the supporting network.

lobe, the veins have a horizontal course as they drain into the left atrium, whereas arteries in the lower lobe lie more vertically. The vertical descending veins in the upper lobe add to the density of the upper portions of the hila, whereas the veins in the lower lobe contribute to the density of the lower portions of the hila. On computed tomography (CT), the anatomy of the ostia of the four pulmonary veins draining into the left atrium is of increasing interest to facilitate the radiofrequency ablation of ectopic foci.

On the erect radiograph film, the diameters of the vessels increase from the apices to the bases. The vessels in the first anterior intercostal space should not exceed 3 mm in normal patients. In congestive cardiac failure, upper zone blood diversion (or cephalisation) occurs and becomes evident on the erect film (see page 100). As seen on the normal erect CXR, the vessels to the lower zones appear larger. Most of the ventilation and perfusion occurs in the lower zones. When the person is horizontal, equalisation of the flow occurs, with enlargement of the vessels to the upper zones. Pulmonary circulation values are shown in Table 2.2.

The right basal pulmonary artery has a width of 9–16 mm in males and 9–15 mm in females. If increased in size, it could indicate pulmonary hypertension.

TABLE 2.2 Pulmonary circulation values

Volume	450–600 mL (about 10% of total blood volume)
Mean arterial pressure	15 mmHg
Mean venous pressure	5 mmHg
Flow at rest	5 L/min
Flow at maximal exercise	20 L/min
Lung height	30 cm

Fig. 2.5 Pulmonary artery anatomy: (a) digital subtraction angiogram; (b) pulmonary angiogram

(a) A catheter has been introduced from the femoral vein. It passes up the *inferior vena cava* (IVC), across the right atrium, tricuspid valve and right ventricle to the main pulmonary artery.

The digital subtraction technology has helped in showing the anatomical relationship between the aorta and pulmonary arteries.

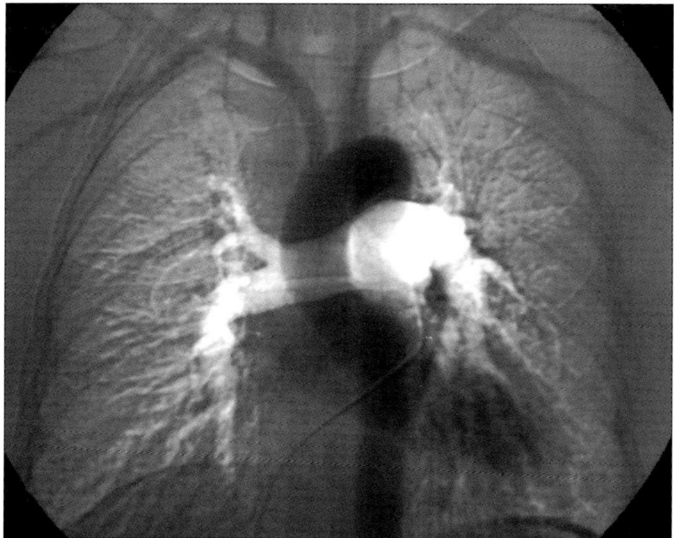

FIG 2.5a

Fig. 2.5 Pulmonary artery anatomy: (a) pulmonary angiogram; (b) digital subtraction angiogram

(b) A catheter has been introduced into the main pulmonary artery via the left arm. The pulmonary arteries have been demonstrated with a contrast injection.

At the right hilum, the right main pulmonary artery is dividing and lying anterior to the right main bronchus. The branches then radiate out into the lung fields.

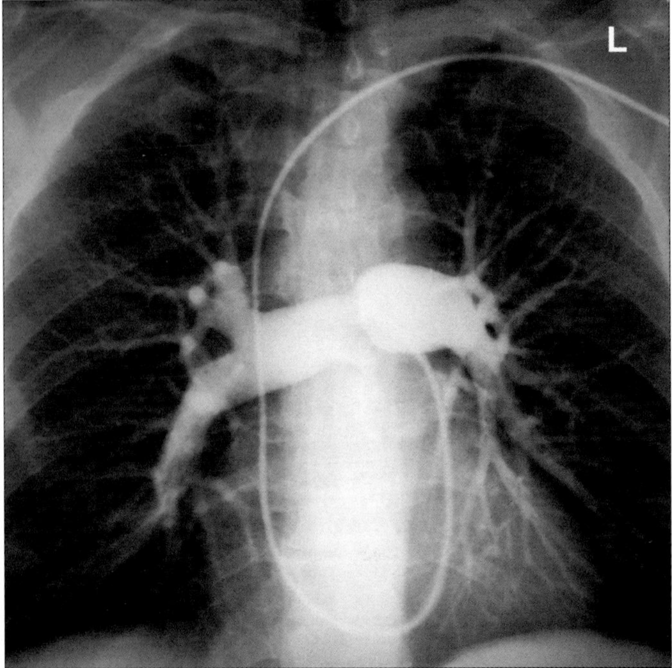

FIG 2.5b

Hila

The hila are the imprecisely defined junctions between the mediastinal structures and the lungs. Their densities are mainly due to the pulmonary arteries but the pulmonary veins, lymph nodes and bronchi also contribute.

The right hilum is in the shape of a V turned on its side and lies 1–2 cm below the height of the left hilum. The left hilum is higher and has a squarer shape.

The critical fact in understanding hilar anatomy is that the left pulmonary artery arches over the left main bronchus to descend posterolateral to the left lower lobe bronchus, whereas the right pulmonary artery passes anterior to the main bronchus and intermediate bronchus, with early origin of the right upper lobe artery at the hilum.

Pleura

The pleurae are smooth thin serous membranes with a single surface layer of mesothelial cells. Deep to the mesothelial cell layer is a fat-containing layer of connective tissue which either connects to the overlying chest wall or underlying lung. The parietal pleura lines the mediastinum (mediastinal pleura) and diaphragm (diaphragmatic pleura) and the inside of the chest wall. The visceral pleura covers the lung. It invaginates into the lungs as two layers to form the fissures. The exception is the azygos fissure which has four layers of pleura.

The parietal and visceral pleura are in continuity as they are reflected around the hilum. Normally, there is only a potential space between the two although it is filled with about 5 mls of lubricating pleural fluid. The two pleural spaces are not connected.

Inferior to the hilum, a double fold of pleura forms the 'inferior pulmonary ligament', connecting the medial aspect of the lower lobe to the mediastinum.

Diaphragm

The diaphragm is a musculotendinous structure that separates the thoracic and abdominal cavities. The peripheral muscular insertions are the crura, ribs 7–12 and the xiphisternum. On each side the muscular fibres converge to the central tendon to form a domed structure. Towards the midline there are three hiati connecting the thoracic and abdominal cavities. Accompanying the aorta through the aortic hiatus is the azygos vein, hemiazygos vein and the thoracic duct. The oesophagus, vagus nerves and paraoesophageal vessels pass through the oesophageal hiatus. The highest and most anterior hiatus is for the IVC to enter the right atrium. The anterior foramina of Morgagni and the posterior foramina of Bochdalek are potential sites of herniation.

The hemidiaphragms are outlined by the aerated lung except on the lateral CXR where the anterior portion is obscured by the heart. The height of the curve is about 2.5 cm.

On the inspiratory frontal film, the apex of the hemidiaphragm should pass as low as the sixth costal cartilage level or the tenth to eleventh rib posteriorly. In thin young athletic patients, the level of the diaphragm will pass more inferiorly and should not be interpreted as 'overinflation'.

The right hemidiaphragm is 2 cm higher than the left in most patients. In 10% of patients the two domes lie at the same level. In 1% the left hemidiaphragm can be slightly higher than the right.

In the posteroanterior (PA) projection, the posterior lung base is hidden below the dome of the diaphragm. The lateral film shows the hemidiaphragms as well as the whole of the lung bases, including the posterior costophrenic angles.

Mediastinum

The mediastinum separates the two pleural cavities and lungs, extending from the cervicothoracic junction above to the diaphragm below, and from the sternum in front to the vertebral column behind. It contains a number of structures, including the heart, great vessels, trachea, oesophagus, lymph nodes, thoracic duct and mediastinal fat. Figure 2.6 shows the margins of the mediastinum.

The aortic knuckle is the junction of the aortic arch and descending aorta. It produces a characteristic configuration above the hilum on the left margin of the superior mediastinum where it is outlined by the apicoposterior segment of the left upper lobe.

The thymus is relatively large in the first three years, filling much of the anterior mediastinal space. It is visible as a mediastinal structure on the frontal CXR up to about 8 years of age (see sail sign, Appendix 2 and Fig 2.6). Although growing slightly until puberty, it becomes relatively smaller, then after the teen years it atrophies and undergoes fatty replacement. The thymus maintains cell-mediated immune responses by producing T lymphocytes.

On each side a phrenic nerve, formed in the neck (C3–5), courses downwards over the lateral wall of the mediastinum, passing anterior to the hilum to reach and supply the hemidiaphragm. Mostly there

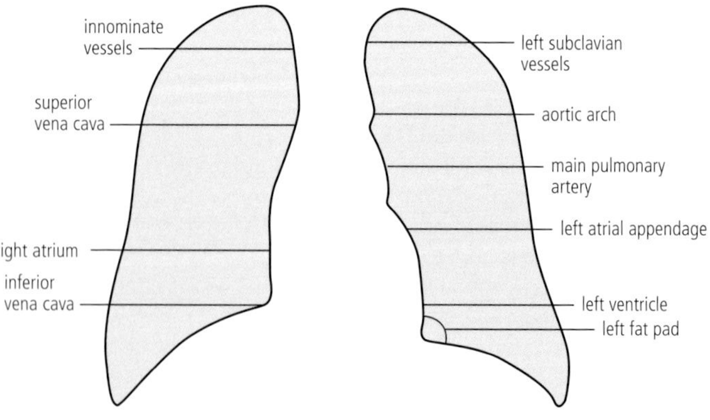

Fig. 2.6 Lateral margins of the mediastinum

are motor nerve fibres to produce the muscular contractions. Injury to the phrenic nerve will cause a unilateral palsy with hemidiaphragm elevation and paradoxical movement on sniffing. The less numerous sensory fibres, if irritated, can cause 'referred' pain to the shoulder.

Mediastinal spaces

The *pretracheal space* is explored by surgeons in transcervical mediastinoscopy in the diagnostic work-up of bronchogenic carcinoma. Lymph nodes here are amenable to biopsy. Remember that 17% of normal-appearing lymph nodes in this space may have microscopic metastases.

The *superior pericardial recess* lies behind the ascending aorta and can mimic lymphadenopathy or aortic dissection.

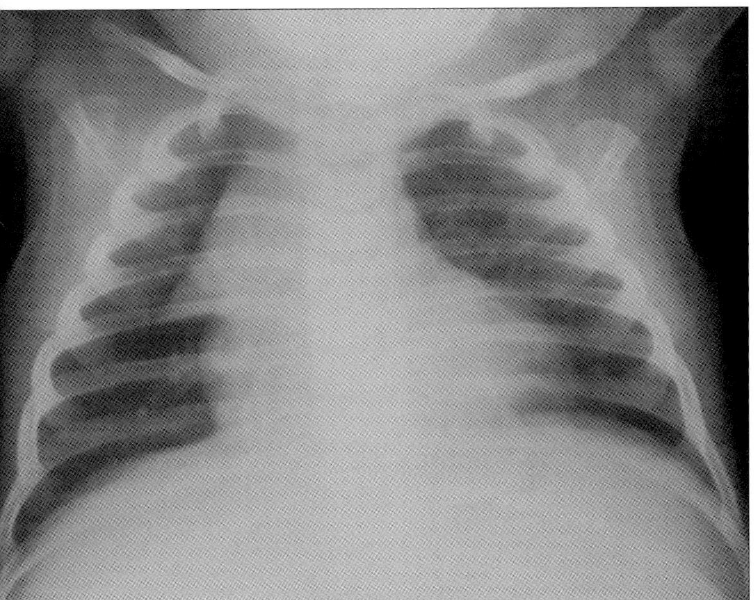

Fig. 2.7 Thymus in a neonate: PA view

In the normal neonate, the thymus often causes a triangular sail shadow, usually on the right upper mediastinum. It needs to be recognised as different from right upper lobe consolidation by its well-defined vertical lateral border; its sharp inferior angle is not seen in encapsulated pleural effusion.

Besides this sail sign, other signs to distinguish the thymus are the 'spinnaker' sign (see Appendix 2) and the thymic 'wave' sign (see Appendix 2).

The thymus swells with crying, the Valsalva manoeuvre and after illness. It shrinks with steroid medication, radiation treatment and during illness.

The *aortopulmonary window* lies between the aortic arch above and the left pulmonary artery below. It contains the ligamentum arteriosum and the recurrent laryngeal nerve. Lymphadenopathy here can cause a left recurrent laryngeal nerve palsy.

The *retrocrural space* is the lower part of the mediastinum behind the diaphragmatic crura. Here the descending aorta leaves the chest, and the azygos and hemiazygos veins are the direct continuation of the upper lumbar veins. The thoracic duct formed from the cisterna chyli also enters the chest.

Interface line, stripes and edges

The lateral edges of the mediastinum are depicted in Fig. 2.6. They are visible because of the interface with the adjacent aerated lung. There are other interfaces where the X-ray beam passes tangentially to an edge of soft tissue adjacent to lung. These radiographic landmarks can help in detecting abnormalities.

A line is a longitudinal opacity no greater than 2 mm in width; a stripe is a longitudinal opacity 2–5 mm in width. These must be distinguished from the Mach effect, which is an optical illusion that can highlight these interfaces. For example, the left heart border can have a dark stripe paralleling its edge and mimicking pneumomediastinum or pneumothorax (negative Mach effect).

The right paratracheal stripe is visible where the right lung abuts the right wall of the trachea. The paravertebral stripes, sometimes called 'paraspinal lines', are sometimes visualised on well-penetrated CXRs. Similarly, the left wall of the descending aorta will show as an interface edge against the aerated adjacent lung. It may produce a para-aortic white stripe (positive Mach effect).

In the majority of patients the lungs are separated by mediastinal fat. However, if the lungs appose (4 layers of pleura) without any intervening mediastinal fat, anterior and posterior junction lines may be visible.

A similar effect occurs to produce the companion shadow of the second rib. The apical pleura appears in profile as a stripe paralleling the inferior border of the posterior aspect of the second rib.

Heart

The anatomy of the margins and configuration of the characteristic cardiovascular silhouette need to be understood so that abnormalities can be detected.

One-third of the heart lies to the right of the midline and two-thirds to the left, with the cardiac apex pointing downwards and outwards to produce the characteristic shape. In the normal adult, the transverse diameter of the cardiac silhouette is less than half the thoracic diameter.

In the frontal projection (see Fig. 2.8), the right heart border is made up entirely by the right lateral margin of the right atrium; the right heart border is outlined by the adjacent aerated medial segment of the middle lobe. The left border of the cardiovascular silhouette has four protuberances—the aortic knob, pulmonary artery, left atrial appendage and left ventricle (from top downwards). The left heart border is formed by the left ventricle margin silhouetted by the aerated lingular segments of the left upper lobe.

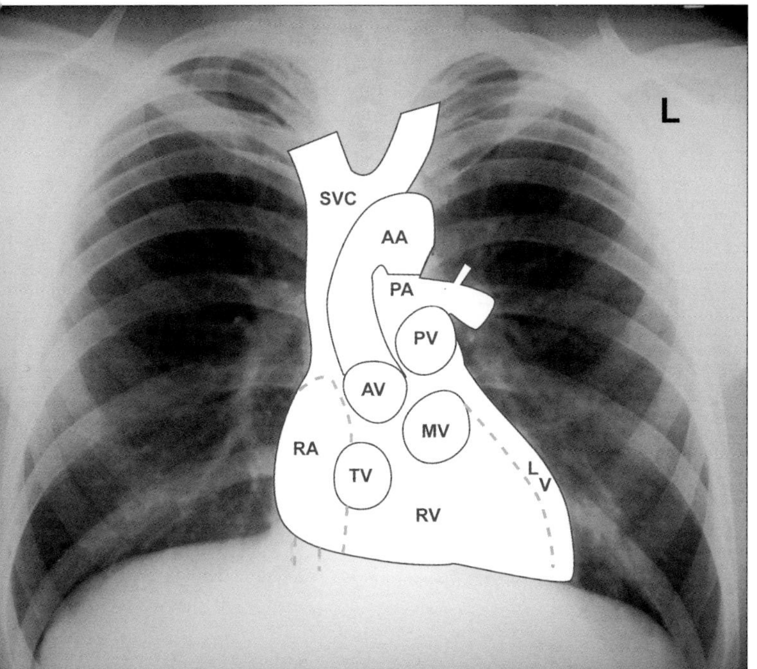

Fig. 2.8 Heart anatomy: frontal projection

The right heart border is formed by the right atrium (RA) with the right mediastinal border formed by the SVC.

The left ventricle (LV) forms the left heart border. The left margin of the right ventricle (RV) is about a finger's breadth in from the left heart border, corresponding to the anterior interventricular groove.

From above downwards, the heart valves are the pulmonary valve (PV), aortic valve (AV), mitral valve (MV) and tricuspid valve (TV).

Within the mediastinum, the main pulmonary artery (PA) lies to the left of the ascending aorta (AA).

The anterior margin of the heart on the lateral CXR (see Fig. 2.9) is formed by the front wall of the right ventricle; the main pulmonary artery and ascending aorta lie above.

The posterior margin of the heart is formed by the posterior margin of the left atrium.

The pericardium surrounds the heart similar to the pleura around the lungs. The visceral pericardium is attached to the myocardium. The parietal pericardium is a thick fibrous layer that blends with adventitia of great vessels as they enter and exit the heart. Within the pericardial sac is about 20 mls of serous fluid for lubrication during cardiac motion.

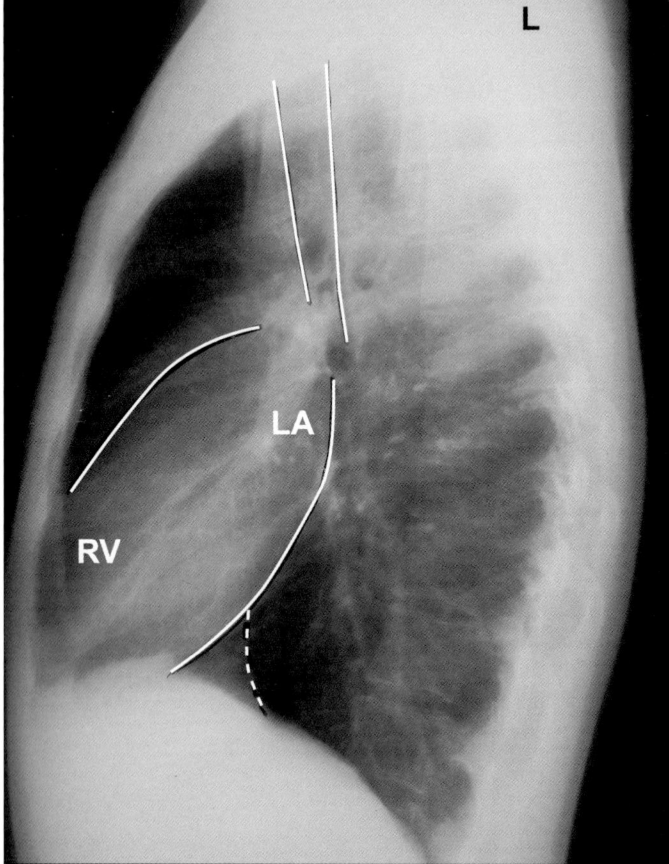

FIG 2.9a

Because of the attachment of the pericardium to the diaphragm, the heart elongates during inspiration and flattens during expiration.

The 'great vessels' is a collective term referring to the major blood vessels attached to the heart. All the vessels have anatomical importance in chest radiology (see Table 2.3, page 28).

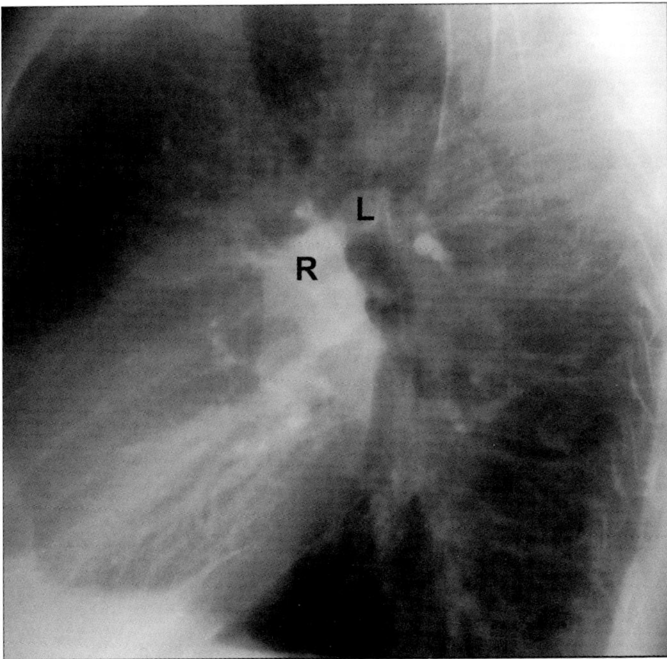

FIG 2.9b

Fig. 2.9 Heart anatomy: (a) lateral view; (b) localised lateral view

(a) The cardiac margins and trachea have been highlighted. The anterior margin of the heart is the right ventricle (RV); the posterior margin is the left atrium (LA). The retrosternal and retrocardiac airspaces should have a similar radiotranslucency. Both hemidiaphragms are visualised and both costophrenic angles are sharp. The lower vertebral bodies are overlaid by an increasing amount of translucent lung.

(b) The trachea can be followed downwards and the lower part of the air column is the major bronchi. The rounded lucency is the upper left lobe bronchus seen end-on.

The left pulmonary artery (L) curves over the left main bronchus. The right pulmonary artery (R) is projected as a circular opacity anterior to the airway.

TABLE 2.3 Great vessels

Venae cavae
• SVC • IVC
Pulmonary arteries
• Pulmonary trunk • Right pulmonary artery • Left pulmonary artery
Pulmonary veins
• Right superior • Left superior • Right inferior • Left inferior
Aorta
Five vessels above aortic arch
• Right brachiocephalic artery • Right brachiocephalic vein • Left common carotid artery • Left brachiocephalic vein • Left subclavian artery

Lymphatic drainage

In the secondary pulmonary lobule, lymphatic vessels are seen accompanying the veins in the interlobular septa and also accompanying the bronchoarterial bundle centrally. These lymphatic vessels converge to form a deep network accompanying the blood vessels and bronchi towards the bronchopulmonary lymph nodes at the hila. There is also a superficial plexus, which drains the visceral pleura and subpleural lung, which also passes to the bronchopulmonary lymph nodes.

Flow is then via tracheobronchial and paratracheal lymph nodes into bronchomediastinal trunks, which either join the right jugular lymph trunk or thoracic duct or enter independently into the brachiocephalic veins. At their terminations they may communicate with scalene lymph nodes.

The exception to the 'homolateral' drainage of the lungs is the left lower lobe and lingula, where the flow passes from the left bronchopulmonary lymph nodes to the carinal lymph nodes and then along the right lymphatic route.

Thoracic duct

The thoracic duct is a component of the posterior mediastinum. It arises from the cisterna chyli, passes into the thoracic cavity through the aortic hiatus, and courses to the right side of the spine between the aorta and azygos vein. At the level of the carina, it swings to the left and ascends along the lateral aspect of the oesophagus and then arches forward to drain into the venous system at the junction of the left innominate and internal jugular veins.

Injury to the lower thoracic duct will cause a right chylothorax whereas higher injury will cause a left chylothorax.

Bones

The density of the bones can hide the fine detail of the lungs. On a good CXR, the radiographer has positioned the patient's arm to rotate the scapulae away from being projected over the lung fields.

The lung apices do not lie higher than the posterior aspects of the first ribs but this is higher than the level of the first costal cartilages. The fronts of the apices, above the clavicles, are therefore exposed to possible injury (e.g. iatrogenic pneumothorax from inadvertent needle puncture).

The second costal cartilage joins the sternum at the manubriosternal junction (about the lower T4 level).

Soft tissues

The thickness of the soft tissue on the chest wall varies depending on the size of the patient. In female patients, the breasts project increased density over the lower zones. In male patients and small-breasted female patients, beware of nipple shadows projected over the lower zones being misinterpreted as nodules.

CHAPTER 3

CHEST X-RAY INTERPRETATION

The best way to inspect a chest radiograph is with a good viewing box (or monitor) and in calm surroundings. An additional bright light should be available for inspecting any dark areas of the film.

Novices can reduce the chance of missing an abnormality by having a directed systematic search pattern rather than a free global search. A checklist is shown in Table 3.1.

SYSTEMATIC SEARCH PATTERN

Documentation

The film should record the patient's name, date and where it was taken. The radiographer should indicate on the film the patient's side and any change from the normal technique (i.e. anteroposterior [AP], mobile, supine, expiratory).

Technique

The film reader needs to be aware of the technique used for proper interpretation (e.g. assessment of heart size will not be valid on an AP film). Poor film centring, incorrect exposure or rotation will produce a less than ideal film and limit the diagnostic information.

Upper mediastinum

The mediastinum appears as a number of structures superimposed on one another.

- The trachea should be of uniform calibre. It enters the thoracic inlet in the middle and passes slightly to the right as it passes the aortic arch.

It may be displaced or compressed by a goitre or lymphadenopathy. An obstructing tracheal tumour could cause dyspnoea or a wheeze.

- The aortic knuckle is reduced in coarctation (see Fig. 3.1) and intracardiac left-to-right shunts. It is not reduced in patent ductus arteriosus (PDA). The aortic knuckle is widened if this portion becomes aneurysmal.
- If the patient is old, the loss of elastic tissue in the aortic walls causes 'unfolding' of the aorta with a more prominent curve. The right lateral margin of the superior mediastinum may be due to the ascending aorta rather than the SVC. (Compare this to the normal anatomy in Fig 2.8.) A similar prominence of the ascending aorta may be seen with post-stenotic dilation in aortic stenosis (AS).

Look for any changes in the outline or width of the superior mediastinum that could indicate that a mass is present. The commonest cause of a widened mediastinum is ectasia or unfolding of the aortic arch and innominate artery with ageing due to the loss of elastic tissue. Mediastinal tumours are discussed in Chapter 7.

TABLE 3.1 Checklist for scrutiny of a chest radiograph

Frontal	Lateral
• Patient name and date	• Patient name and date
• Technique	• Technique
• Upper mediastinum including trachea	• Trachea
• Hila	• Hilar density and main pulmonary arteries
• Heart	• Heart and great vessels
• Diaphragm and below	• Diaphragm and below
• Lung fields: Check margins Compare zones	• Pleural fissures: Retrosternal space Retrocardiac space Posterior costophrenic angles
• Bones	• Thoracic spine, ribs
• Soft tissues	• Soft tissues
• Overall review	• Overall review
• Check for pneumothorax	
• Are there previous films for comparison?	

Remember that the superior mediastinum, including the trachea and the heart, will be shifted *towards* a collapsed lung and *away* from a large pleural effusion (see Fig. 3.2) or tension pneumothorax (see Fig. 6.1).

Fig. 3.1 Aortic coarctation: PA view

Coarctation of the aorta is a congenital short segment narrowing of the distal aortic arch just beyond the origin of the left subclavian artery; at or just beyond, the ligamentum arteriosum.

The plain film shows the small appearing aortic knuckle. Sometimes the left paravertebral shadow is widened due to the hypertrophied left subclavian artery.

If a barium swallow is performed, the oesophagus is identified by the dilated portions of the aorta just proximal and just distal to the coarctation.

Inferior notching of the adult fourth to eighth ribs is sometimes more easily seen than the aortic abnormalities. The notching is from the pulsatile retrograde flow in the dilated intercostal arteries supplying blood to the descending aorta.

Possible associated abnormalities are congenital heart disease, including bicuspid aortic valve, intracranial berry aneurysms and Turner's syndrome. (See differential diagnosis of inferior rib notching, Appendix 3).

Fig. 3.2 Pleural effusion: PA view

A large, left pleural effusion is present causing a homogeneous opacity with a characteristic concave upper margin of meniscus shape. The underlying lung will be passively collapsed with more blood being delivered into the right pulmonary circulation. There is mediastinal shift to the right with the left heart border obscured. Inversion of the left hemidiaphragm has produced displacement of the gastric gas shadow.

Remember that different fluids, such as transudates or exudates, will have similar appearances because of their similar X-ray density. The actual cause of the effusion may need to be established from the history, other clinical or radiological findings or analysis of the aspirate itself. The common causes of unilateral pleural effusion are infection, tumour—either primary or secondary—haemorrhage or chylothorax.

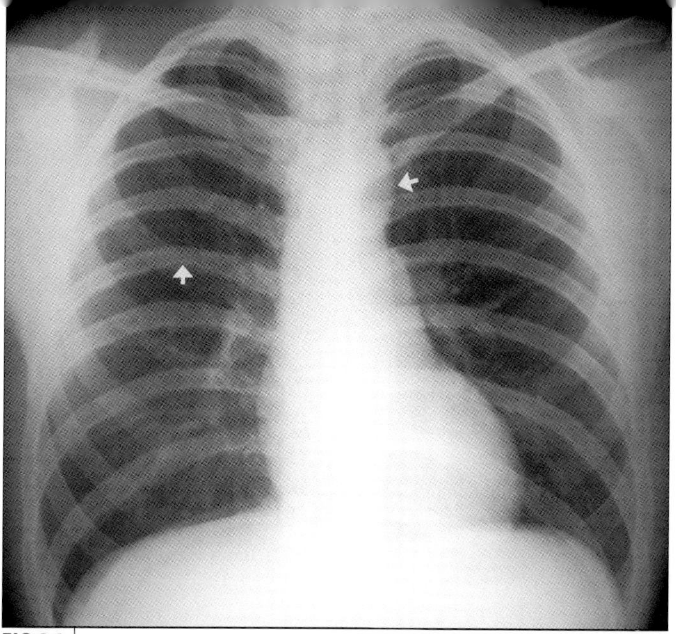

FIG 3.1

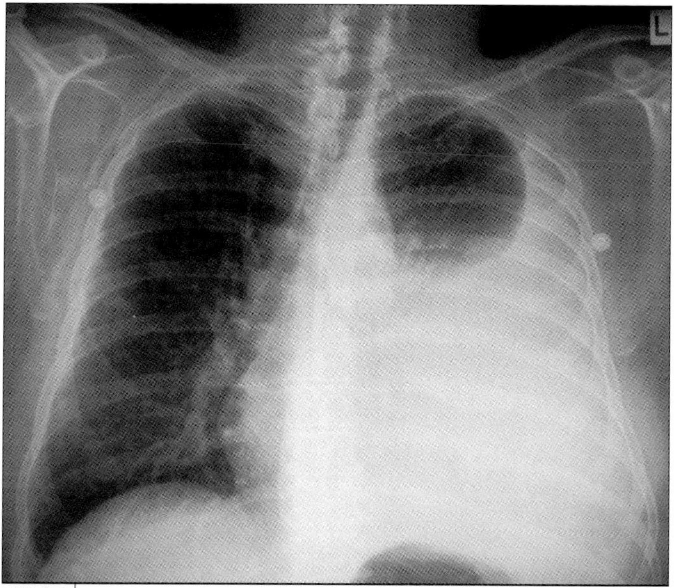

FIG 3.2

Hila

The left hilum will be 1–2 cm higher than the right hilum mainly because the left main pulmonary artery passes up and over the left main bronchus. The right hilum has a V-shape, with the left hilum being squarer. Even though there is a difference in the positions and shapes, the hila should have the same density. A dense hilum could be due to a lymphadenopathy or an adjacent confluent mass.

When hilar lymphadenopathy is present, it is important to distinguish between lymphadenopathy and arteriomegaly. Scrutinise the film to see if there are other sites of lymphadenopathy or whether there are prominent vessels just outside the hilum (see Fig. 3.3). The vascular causes of enlarged hila are pulmonary hypertension seen in left-to-right shunts, emphysema (see Fig. 3.4) and chronic pulmonary emboli. A hilum may appear prominent when a large acute embolus is present (see Fleischner sign, Appendix 2).

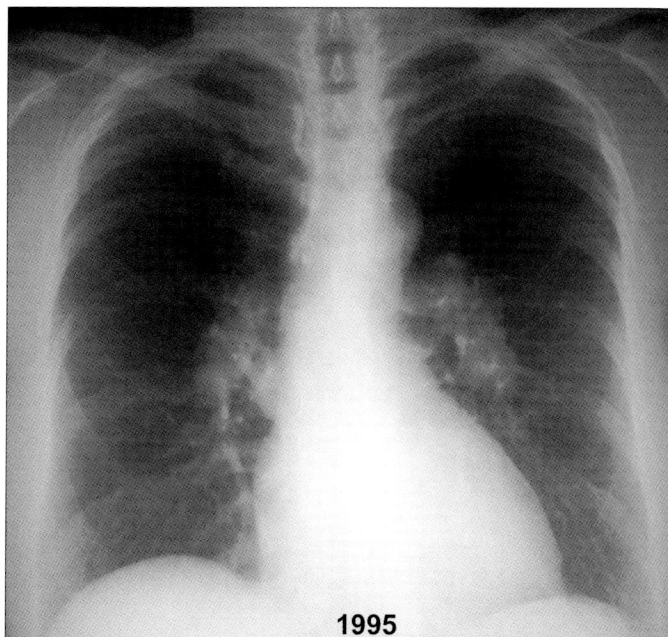

FIG 3.3a

Fig. 3.3 Bilateral hilar lymphadenopathy: (a) PA view; (b) PA view; (c) lateral view

The first interpretative decision to make when enlarged hila are recognised is whether the hilar enlargement is due to lymphadenopathy or enlarged pulmonary arteries.

(a) The 1995 CXR shows a 'clear space' between the hilum and the mediastinum. This floating hilum sign (see Appendix 2) distinguishes hilar lymphadenopathy from mediastinal lymphadenopathy.

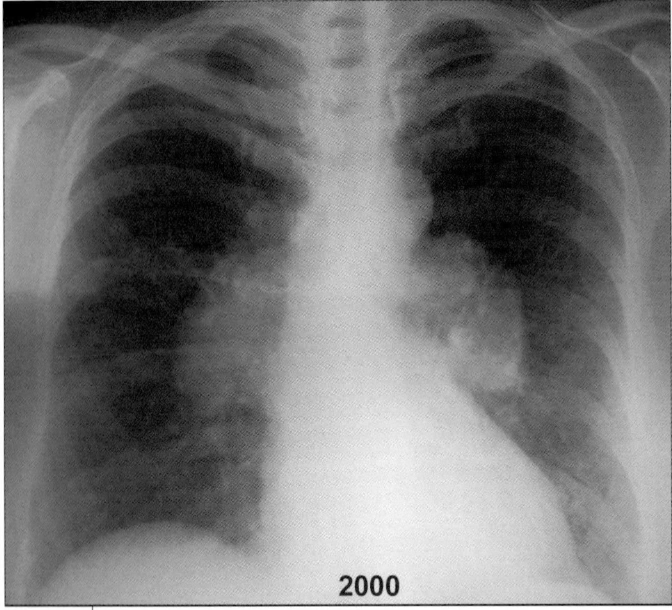

FIG 3.3b

Fig. 3.3 Bilateral hilar lymphadenopathy: (a) PA view; (b) PA view; (c) lateral view

(b) By 2000, the hilar lymphadenopathy has further increased.

(c) This lateral view also shows the hilar lymphadenopathy.

Hilar symmetry is unusual in the major alternative diagnoses of lymphoma, tuberculosis and metastases. (See differential diagnosis of hilar lymphadenopathy, Appendix 3.)

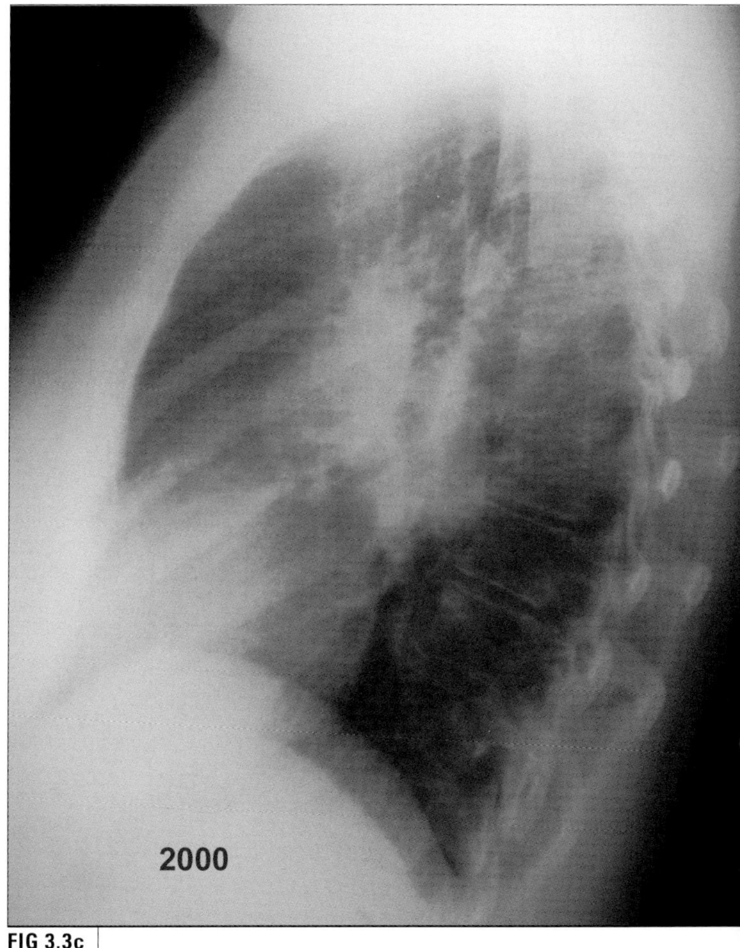

FIG 3.3c

Heart

Two-thirds of the heart lies to the left of the midline with the bulk of the heart projected over the left lower zone. Fat pads may blunt the cardiophrenic angles. The heart borders (see Fig. 3.5) should be sharp. If not, the adjacent lung could be consolidated or collapsed (see silhouette sign, Appendix 2). The right heart border may be absent in pectus excavatum.

Enlargement of the right atrium causes the right heart border to bulge. Marked deviation and enlargement is seen with Ebstein's anomaly.

Right ventricular enlargement produces a cardiac apex that points upwards and outwards on the frontal film (e.g. *cœur en sabot* shape in tetralogy of Fallot). The right ventricle forms the anterior cardiac margin and, with enlargement, more of the anterior margin bulges against the sternum.

Left atrial enlargement causes a bulge of the posterior cardiac margin. In the past this was confirmed by the lateral barium swallow view showing the indentation on the oesophagus. Nowadays, it is confirmed by echocardiography.

The left atrial appendage enlarges with left atrial enlargement and can produce the third mogul (first mogul is the aortic arch, second mogul is the pulmonary artery at the left hilum).

The left ventricle is the major cardiac chamber. As it enlarges the cardiac shadow generally enlarges and the apex points further outwards and downwards.

A normal-sized heart should have a transverse diameter that is less than 50% of the transthoracic diameter on a posteroanterior (PA) X-ray. Left ventricular hypertrophy does not cause recognisable cardiomegaly on the PA film. It is only in patients with heart failure and ventricular dilatation or those with pericardial effusion that the cardiothoracic ratio will exceed 50%. On AP views, the heart is further away from the film and appears larger, and hence the 50% rule cannot be used in AP X-rays.

Factors that may mimic cardiac enlargement, such as poor inspiration, abdominal distension, pectus excavatum and large fat pads, need to be excluded. If a pericardial effusion is suspected, this is best confirmed by ultrasound. The cardiopericardial silhouette may appear enlarged when a pericardial effusion of more than 250 mls has accumulated.

If the heart is enlarged, look for selective chamber enlargement. A double right heart border may indicate an enlarged left atrium due to mitral valve disease. The right atrium will be selectively enlarged in Ebstein's anomaly.

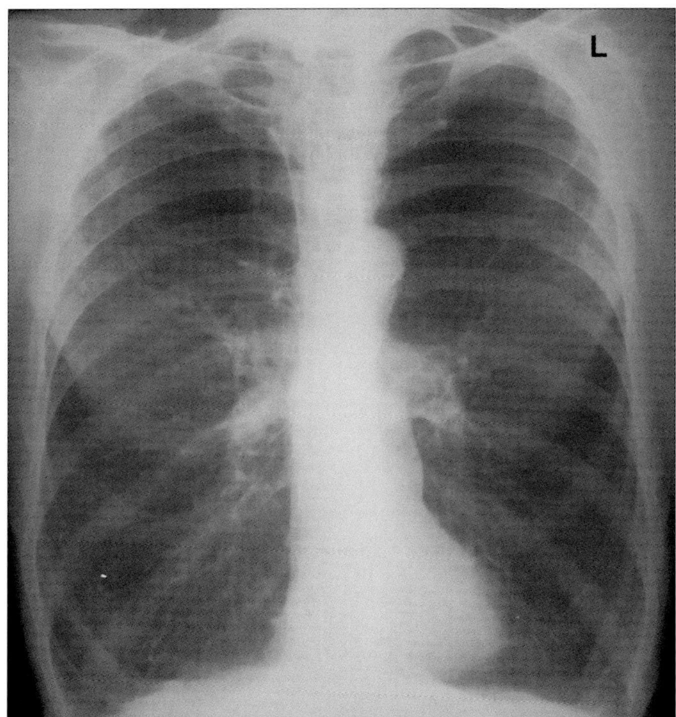

Fig. 3.4 Emphysema: PA view

Emphysema is defined as a lung disease characterised by abnormal permanent enlargement of the air spaces distal to the terminal bronchiole. There is accompanying destruction of the distal air space walls without fibrosis and also loss of the local elastic network.

This radiograph of a case of severe emphysema shows the classic features of overinflation, oligaemia, parenchymal lung destruction and bullae formation. The resultant pulmonary hypertension is reflected in the prominence of the central pulmonary arteries. A 'hanging drop heart' may be another sign.

The lateral CXR would show an increase in the AP diameter of the chest, an increase in the retrosternal airspace and flattening of the hemidiaphragms.

Key points:

- CXR is insensitive for mild and moderate emphysema.
- CXR reliably detects severe emphysema and can be used to exclude severe disease.
- Over-inflation needs to be assessed in regard to age and body habitus.
- Other causes of chronic obstructive pulmonary disease (COPD) are chronic bronchitis, bronchiolitis obliterans and asthma.

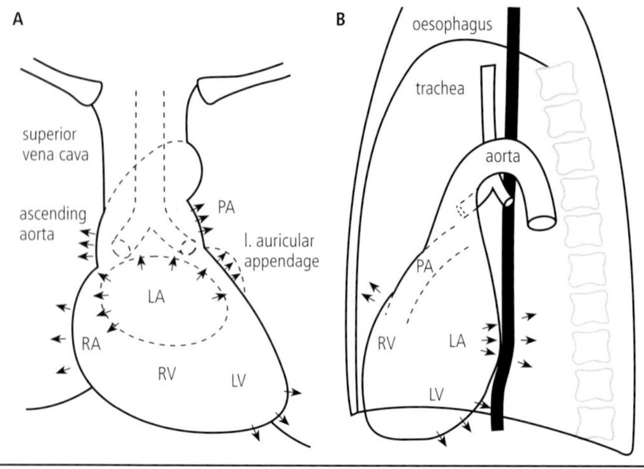

Fig. 3.5 The cardiac borders change with selective chamber enlargement
The arrows indicate the different directions with the enlargement of different chambers (RA=right atrium; RV=right ventricle; LA=left atrium; LV=left ventricle; PA=pulmonary artery). Reproduced with kind permission of Professor WSC Hare from *Clinical Radiology for Medical Students and Health Practitioners*, 2nd ed, Blackwell Science Asia Pty Ltd, 1999.

Calcification of the aortic and mitral valves needs to be sought within the heart shadow. A dense curved or annular calcified band around the mitral valve indicates mitral annulus calcification, which is usually not significant but can cause insufficiency if rigid.

A double density or an air–fluid level behind the heart may suggest a hiatus hernia.

Diaphragm

On the PA X-ray, the hemidiaphragms have convex, smooth upper margins. They represent the highest edge of this curved structure tangential to the X-ray beam. With good inspiration, the apex of each hemidiaphragm should reach the level of the sixth costal cartilage anteriorly and at least the tenth rib posteriorly. The right hemidiaphragm is usually 2 cm higher than the left and has the bulk of the liver beneath it. If the diaphragmatic outline is lost, it means that there is adjacent fluid, consolidation or collapse. Pleural effusions will blunt the costophrenic angles.

In normal patients the height of the hemidiaphragm curve on both the PA and lateral view is about 2 cm. In chronic airways limitation disease the hemidiaphragms will appear flat.

Free gas under the diaphragm seen on erect views usually indicates rupture of a hollow viscus.

Lung fields

The lung fields should be equally translucent. The 'lung markings' are the blood-filled pulmonary vessels and not the bronchi. The pulmonary arteries radiate from the hila; the pulmonary veins radiate into the left atrium.

For convenience, the lung fields on the frontal view are divided into zones. The upper zones are between the lung apices and the level of the second costal cartilages. The mid-zones are between the second and fourth costal cartilage levels, and the lower zones are between the level of the fourth costal cartilage and the diaphragm. The apices lie above the clavicles; the lung bases are the lowest 2 cm.

Compare one side with the other. It is at this time that nodules, consolidation and atelectasis are usually recognised.

Consolidation means that the airspaces are filled with material which replaces the air (see Fig. 3.6). This could be an exudate, transudate, blood, protein or even tumour cells—it can sometimes be difficult to distinguish infection, oedema or infarction as a cause of an opaque lung. Bronchial obstruction by a tumour can cause distal consolidation or collapse. A collapsed lung appears opaque because the air has been lost (it is therefore wrong to call it 'collapse–consolidation') (see Figs. 3.7–3.11).

An 'air bronchogram' sign (see Appendix 2) occurs when air is seen in a bronchus because the surrounding parenchyma is opacified. This is abnormal when seen beyond the second branching of the bronchi. The horizontal fissure is visible in two-thirds of patients as a thin, opaque line at the level of the fourth costal cartilage. It passes on the PA view from the lateral aspect of the sixth rib to the right hilum. The horizontal fissure will be raised in collapse or deflationary change of the right upper lobe.

The commonest lobar collapse is that of the left lower lobe, but it is the one most easily missed. The signs are double density behind the heart, loss of outline of the medial left hemidiaphragm, and 'tucking-in' of the left hilum.

If the heart is enlarged, check for further signs of heart failure and oedema. Possible findings range from pulmonary venous congestion and interstitial oedema to alveolar oedema with pleural effusion.

Scrutinise the edges of the lung fields for any pleural abnormalities—effusion, plaque or calcification. When fluid accumulates in the pleural space it appears opaque and causes passive atelectasis of the adjacent lung. The pleural fluid could be a transudate, exudate, blood or chyle. If the effusion is free, it will show a characteristic meniscus sign on X-rays taken with the patient standing. Remember that some posterior basal lung lies below the apex of the hemidiaphragm on the PA film.

Fig. 3.6 Patterns of lobar consolidation
(a) right upper lobe; **(b)** middle lobe; **(c)** right lower lobe; **(d)** left upper lobe; **(e)** left lower lobe

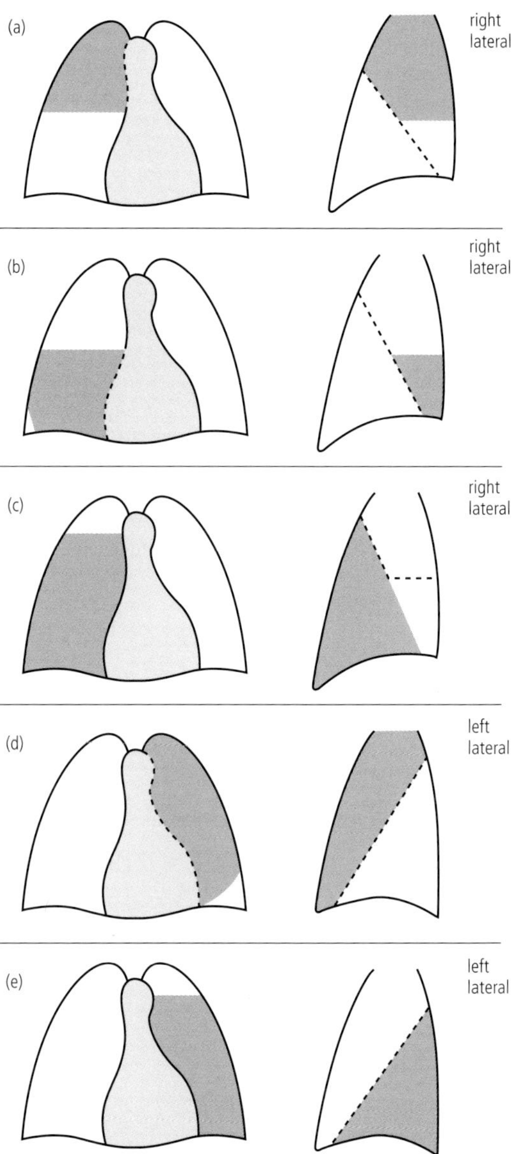
(a)
right lateral
(b)
right lateral
(c)
right lateral
(d)
left lateral
(e)
left lateral

FIG 3.6

Fig. 3.7 Patterns of lobar collapse

(a) Right upper lobe collapse. The horizontal fissure is drawn upwards and the major fissure above the hilum is displaced anteriorly.

(b) Right middle lobe collapse. In both projections, the horizontal fissure is drawn downwards towards the right heart border. The lateral view shows that the lower part of the major fissure is displaced forwards.

(c) Right lower lobe collapse. On the lateral view, the whole of the oblique fissure is displaced backwards. The major fissure is not visible on the PA view until the collapse is almost complete.

(d) Left upper lobe collapse. On the lateral view, the whole of the fissure is displaced upwards and anteriorly. The major fissure does not become visible on the PA projection. There is a band of translucency adjacent to the aortic arch (see luftsichel sign, Appendix 2). Otherwise, loss of translucency is seen in the left upper and mid-zones. Note that there is a major difference in the pattern of collapse between the right upper and left upper lobes.

(e) Left lower lobe collapse. The lateral view shows that the major fissure is displaced posteriorly as in collapse of the right lower lobe. The collapsed lobe is seen as a triangular density projected behind the cardiac shadow. Compensatory overinflation of the left upper lobe occurs with splaying of its pulmonary vessels.

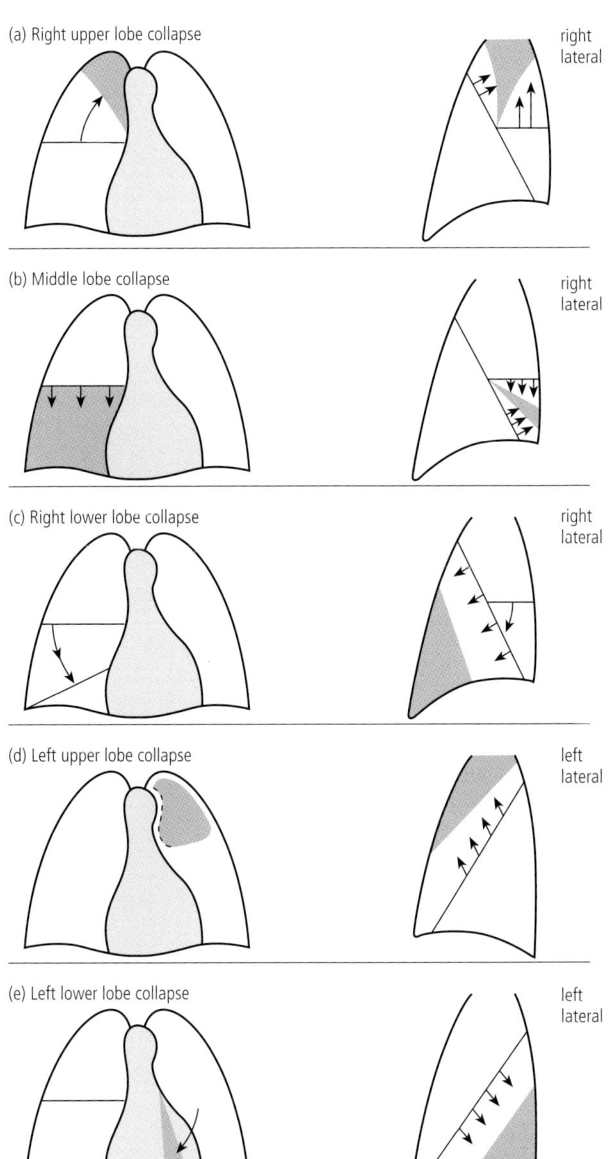
(a) Right upper lobe collapse
right lateral
(b) Middle lobe collapse
right lateral
(c) Right lower lobe collapse
right lateral
(d) Left upper lobe collapse
left lateral
(e) Left lower lobe collapse
left lateral

FIG 3.7

3

Fig. 3.8 Middle lobe collapse: (a) PA view; (b) lateral view

The airless middle lobe lies against the right heart border and has produced loss of the cardiac outline, the so-called 'silhouette sign' (see Appendix 2). Because the middle lobe has a small volume, no recognisable changes are seen in the right hilum or right pulmonary vessels.

On the lateral radiograph there is a wedge-shaped opacity from the horizontal fissure displaced inferiorly and the lower half of the oblique fissure displaced superiorly.

CT scanning or bronchoscopy will be necessary to ascertain whether it is an obstructive atelectasis from a central tumour.

The right middle lobe syndrome is a pattern of recurrent or chronic atelectasis due to extrinsic lymph node compression of the lobar bronchus and poor collateral ventilation.

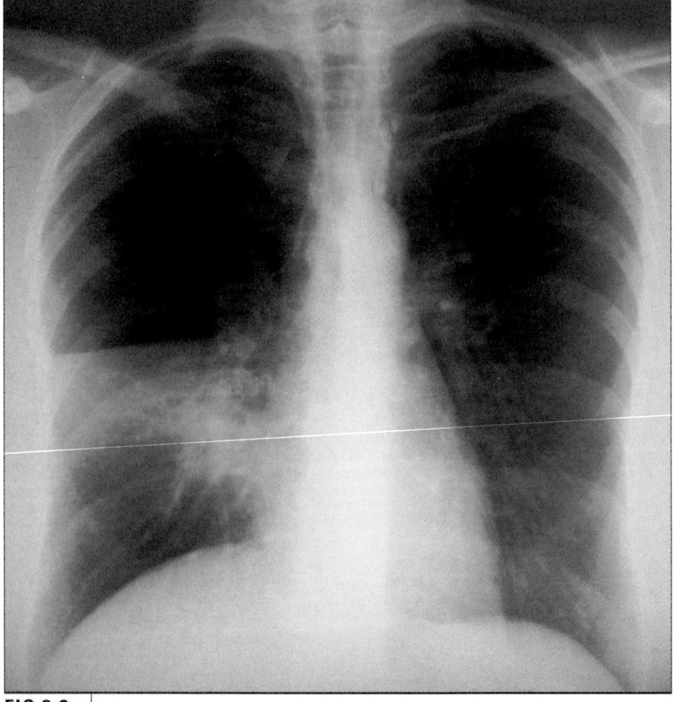

FIG 3.8a

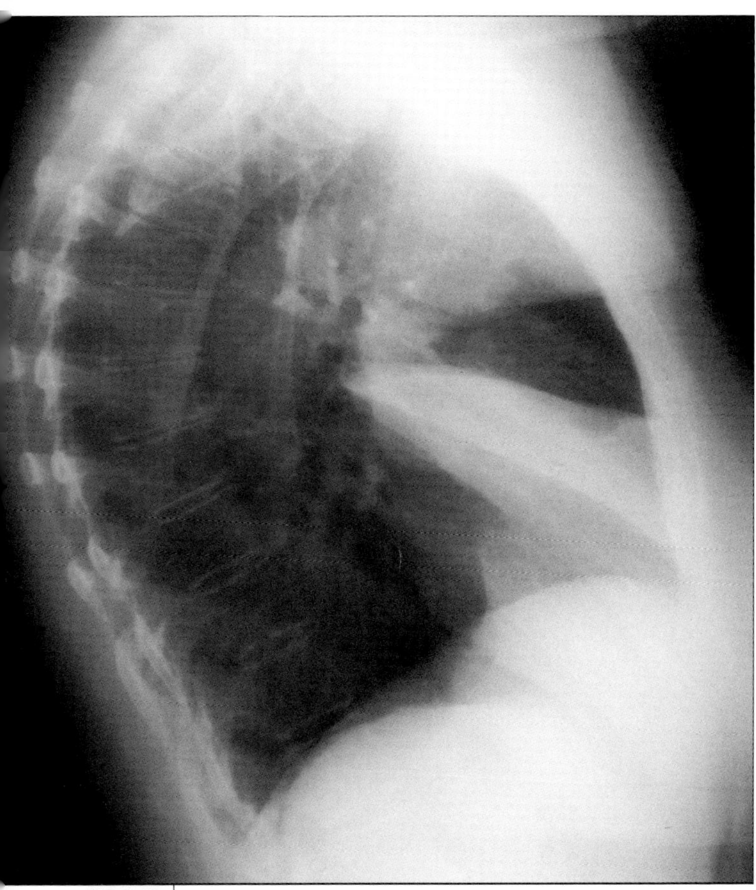

FIG 3.8b

Fig. 3.9 Left lower lobe collapse: (a) lateral view; (b) PA view; (c) CT scan

Left lower lobe collapse is the most common lobar collapse and the most difficult to recognise.

The lobe collapses posteromedially against the posterior mediastinum and spine. On the PA view it appears as a triangular opacity behind the heart and adjacent to the spine (black arrow).

Other signs are the inferior displacement of the left hilum (white arrow), leftward shift of the heart, elevation and poor visualisation of the left hemidiaphragm, and compensatory hyperinflation of the left upper lobe. Also there is flattening of the left cardiac border (see flat waist sign, Appendix 2).

Bronchoscopy is indicated to ascertain the cause for the collapse. Obstructive atelectasis could be due to an endobronchial tumour or an extrinsic mass. In post-operative and ill patients, a mucous plug may be the cause and will need removal.

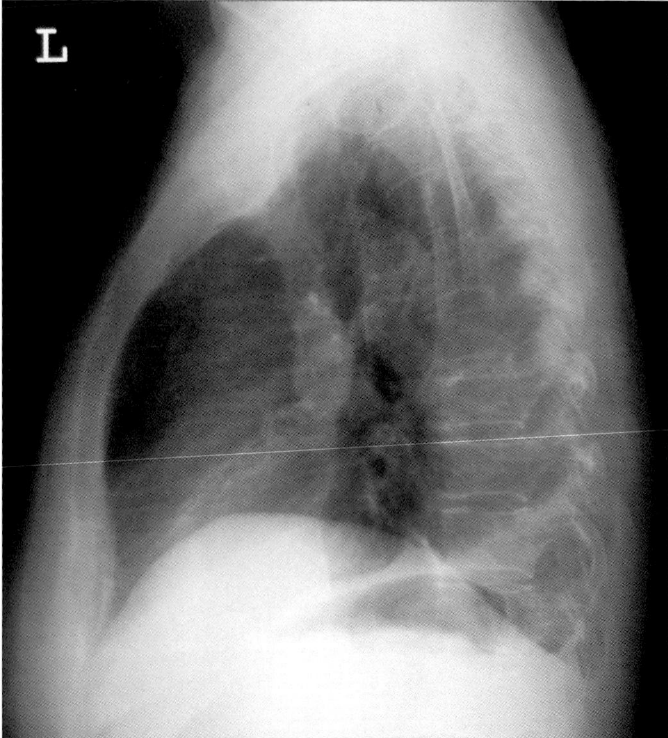

FIG 3.9a

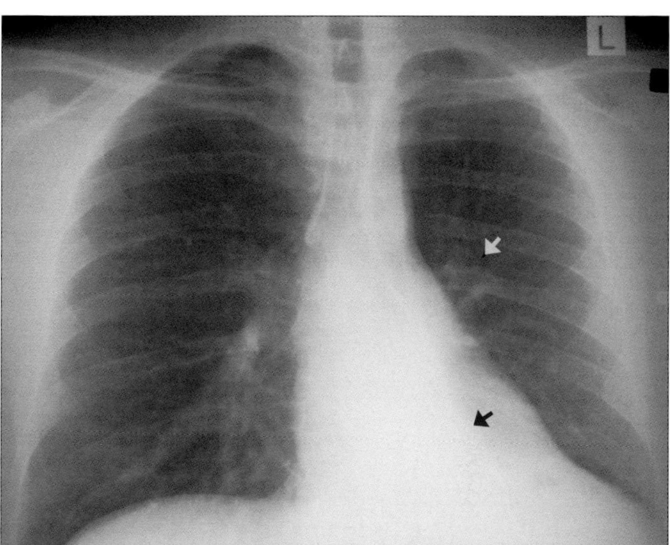

FIG 3.9b

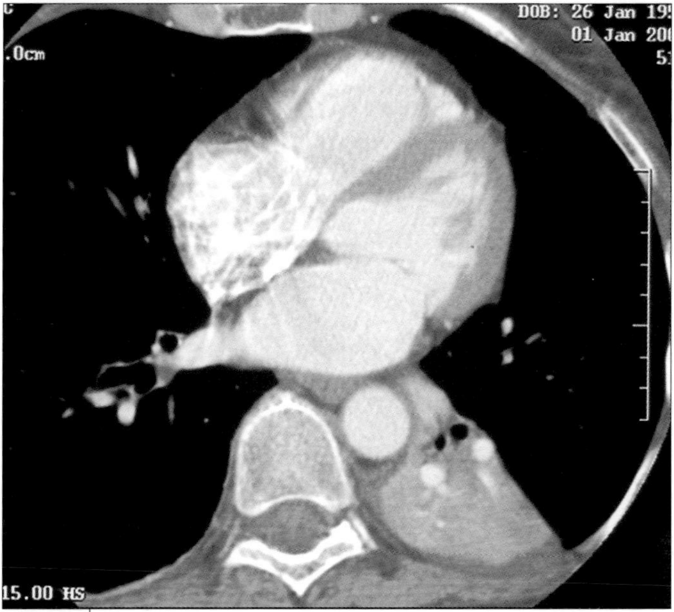

FIG 3.9c

Fig. 3.10 Left upper lobe collapse: (a) PA view; (b) lateral view; (c) CT scan

On the frontal film, there is decreased translucency in the left upper and mid-zones, loss of the left heart border silhouette, leftward superior mediastinal shift, a high position of the left hemidiaphragm and the appearance of the luftsichel sign (see Appendix 2). In addition, there is a left hilar mass indicating that the collapse is due to tumour obstruction of the left upper lobe bronchus (also well shown on the CT scan).

The characteristic forward deviation of the major fissure is seen on the lateral view, with the collapsed lobe seen as a triangular opacity. On the CT scan, note the aerated lung adjacent to the upper part of the descending aorta to help explain the luftsichel sign (see Appendix 2). Herniation of right lung is also seen across the midline, anterior to the ascending aorta, on the CT scan and the lateral view.

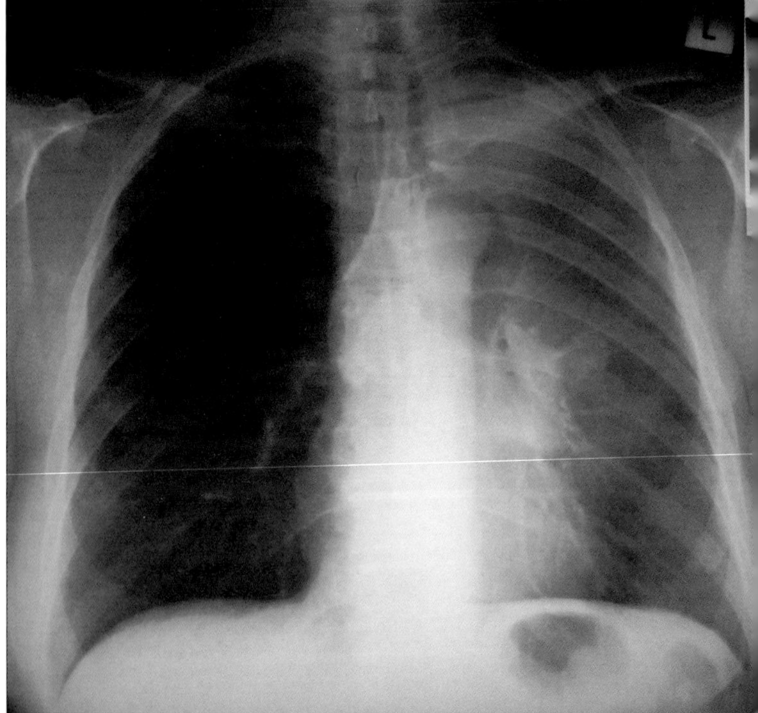

FIG 3.10a

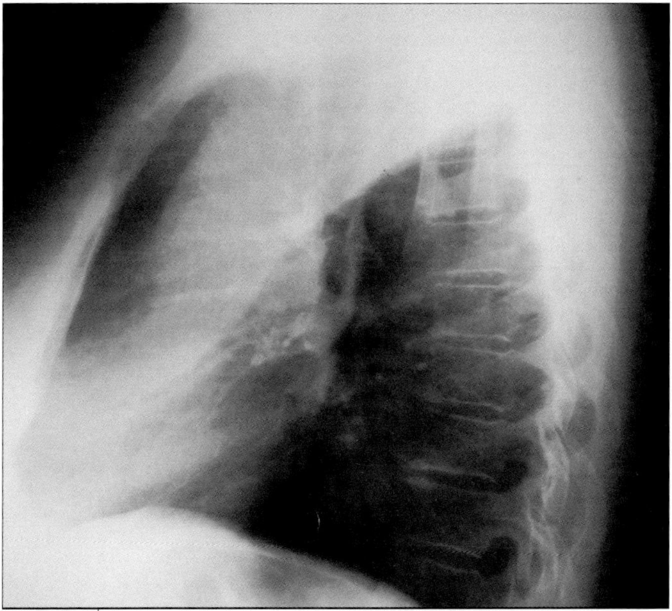

FIG 3.10b

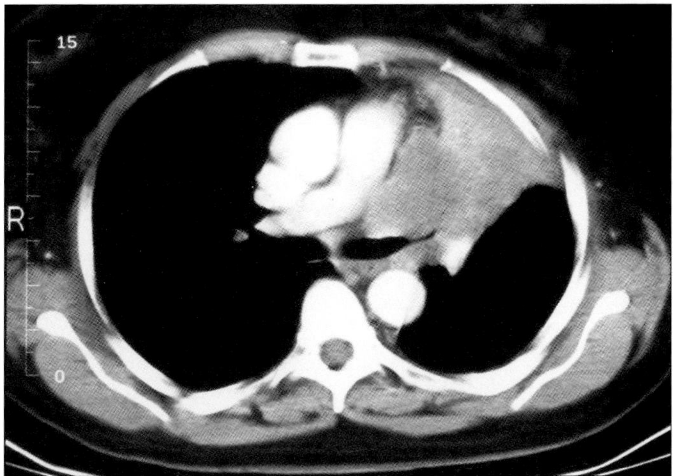

FIG 3.10c

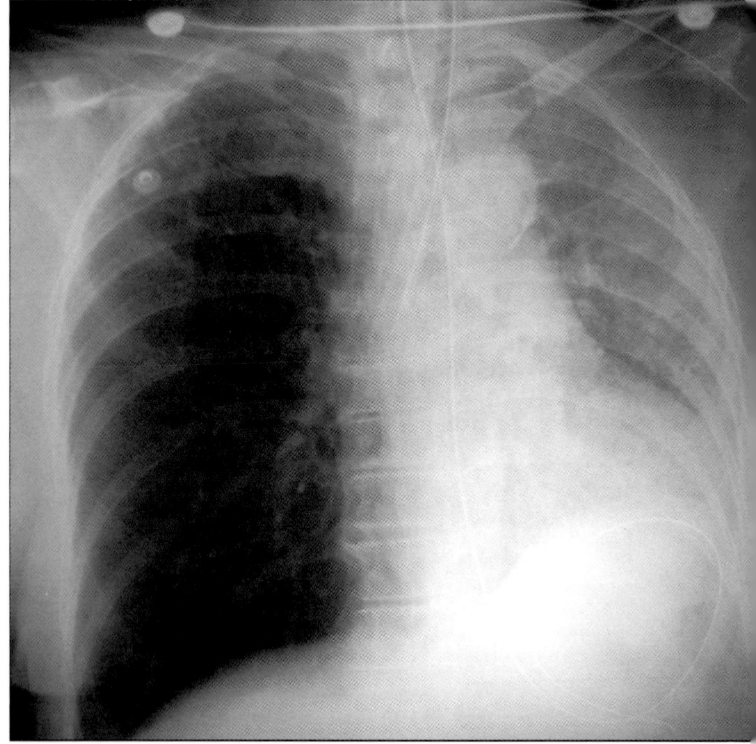

Fig. 3.11 Left lung collapse: PA view

Inadvertent intubation of the right main bronchus has restricted the aeration of the left lung causing incomplete collapse.

The left lung is small with increased opacification, leftward shift of the mediastinum and elevation of the left hemidiaphragm.

The right main bronchus is more vertical in orientation and therefore more likely to be selectively intubated. Sometimes, intubation of the right main bronchus can cause collapse of the right upper lobe as well.

Bones

A quick perusal of the ribs, clavicles, scapulas and lower cervical spine should follow. The ribs and intercostal spaces should have symmetrical widths and shape. If there is a specific concern about rib fractures, then more attention is necessary. Subtle, undisplaced fractures of the lateral ribs are better observed with the film rotated on the viewing box so that the observer can scan the lateral rib edges horizontally.

Inferior rib notching occurs with coarctation of the aorta but there are other causes.

Costal cartilage calcification in elderly patients occurs at the margins in men and centrally in women. Note if a cervical rib is present. Note that scoliosis of the thoracic spine frequently accounts for mediastinal distortions. Look at the paraspinal lines behind the heart and mediastinum. They can be displaced in trauma, infectious spondylodiscitis and posterior mediastinal masses.

Soft tissues

In women, the soft tissues of the breast appear as shadows. Women with large breasts will have increased density over the lower zones. Alternatively, if there has been a mastectomy, the lower zone lung on that side will appear more transradient. Further, radiation fibrosis may explain any upper-zone scarring (see Fig. 3.12).

Soft tissues include those seen below the diaphragm. A CXR may show such abnormalities as calcified hydatid cysts in the liver and splenomegaly (which displaces the gastric air bubble under the left hemidiaphragm). If barium is seen in the bowel, this may be a clue that the patient has another problem which has already been investigated.

Review

A second look at the lung fields partially obscured by the ribs, clavicles and heart is the next step. Most missed lesions lie in the apices, behind the medial ends of the clavicles or behind the left side of the heart. Because the apices are a common site for post-primary tuberculosis, a lordotic AP view may be needed. This will project the clavicles above the apices for better visualisation.

Table 3.2 shows the common pitfalls in interpreting CXRs and Table 3.3 shows false negative causes of CXR interpretation.

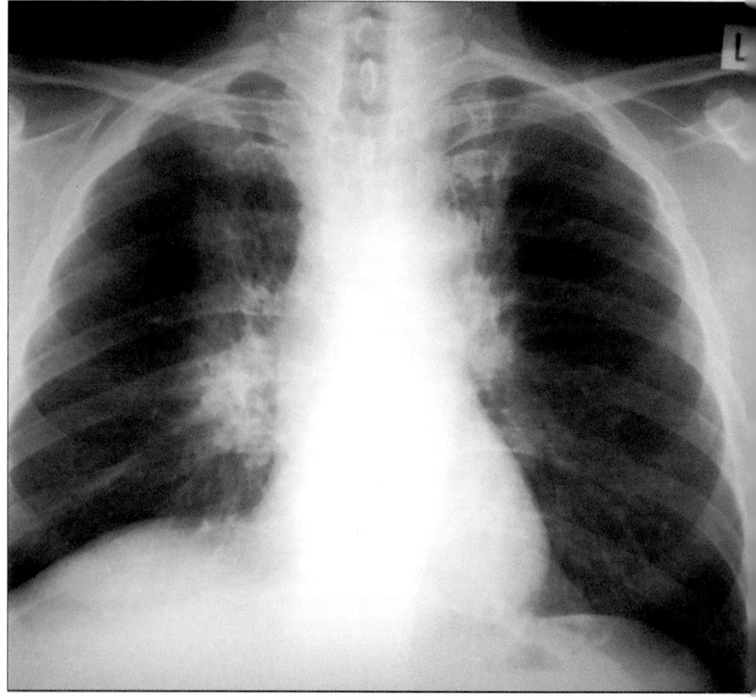

Fig. 3.12 Radiation fibrosis: PA view

Radiation therapy may injure the exposed lung firstly by an acute phase of radiation pneumonitis and then by fibrosis. The sharp lateral borders, as seen in this case, correspond to the radiation ports rather than any anatomical boundary.

The fibrosis is shown as coarse, linear stranding. With further progressive fibrosis, volume loss will occur with elevation of the hila.

TABLE 3.2	Common pitfalls in interpreting chest X-rays
	1. Wrong patient/wrong film/wrong date.
	2. Not recognising a post-mastectomy chest wall in a female patient.
	3. Mistaking costal cartilage calcification in elderly patients for intrathoracic disease.
	4. The lung fields may appear plethoric with crowded markings, the mediastinum widened and the diaphragm elevated in expiratory or supine chest films.
	5. Not recognising skin folds as a cause of an opacity or margin, or confusing a skin fold with a pneumothorax.
	6. Incorrect diagnosis of cardiomegaly on a mobile or anteroposterior film.
	7. Confusing a nipple shadow for a pulmonary nodule (the nipple shadows can be distinguished from other rounded opacities in the lower zones by skin markers).
	8. Not recognising that the loss of elastic tissue in the aorta and main branches results in an 'unfolded aorta', which occurs with age and may mimic paratracheal masses.
	9. Not recognising that pectus excavatum may compress the heart, which then appears as cardiomegaly.
	10. Not recognising spurious 'hilar' lesions where the hilar margins are visible through the opacity (e.g. an apical lesion in the lower lobe projected over the hilum on the frontal film) (see hilum overlay sign, Appendix 2).
	11. Not knowing that extrapleural lipomatosis in obese patients can simulate pleural thickening.

TABLE 3.3	Reasons for false negative chest X-ray interpretation
	• Faulty visual search
	• Satisfaction of search effect (search is terminated after discovery of an abnormality)
	• Faulty pattern recognition
	• Faulty decision making

3

Pneumothorax

In any ordered scrutiny of the CXR film it is worthwhile checking for a small pneumothorax, especially in hospitalised patients. The pneumothorax may be hard to see because the low density of the inflated lung periphery and the free pleural gas are similar (see Fig. 3.13). Beware of missing a pneumothorax on an over-penetrated CXR in which the lung fields are dark.

If a pneumothorax is large, it could be under tension, which is life-threatening for the patient. The signs are:

- the mediastinum is shifted away
- the diaphragm is displaced downwards and the lung is collapsed. These signs are even more dramatic on the expiratory film.

Fig. 3.13 Pneumothorax: PA view

The pleural space is normally a potential space with only a small amount of lubricating pleural fluid present. Pneumothorax literally means free air in the pleural space between the parietal pleura and the visceral pleura. It can be difficult to distinguish density differences between the free air and the peripheral lung where no vascular shadows are present. The pneumothorax is easier to see on expiratory films as the size of the pneumothorax remains constant and the deflated lung becomes denser.

The visceral pleural line (arrowed) is thin.

Even a small pneumothorax is important to identify as it may rapidly increase in size in patients being artificially ventilated. For practical purposes, a pneumothorax can be reported as small, medium or large. Occasionally, clinicians may want an estimation of the pneumothorax size (see Collins CD et al. 'Quantification of pneumothorax size on chest radiographs using interpleural distances'. *AJR* 1995; 165: 1127).

In this case, the 1 cm rim of pneumothorax is occupying about 15–20%. However, the patient's clinical status is more important than the exact percentage of collapse. (See differential diagnosis of pneumothorax, Appendix 3.)

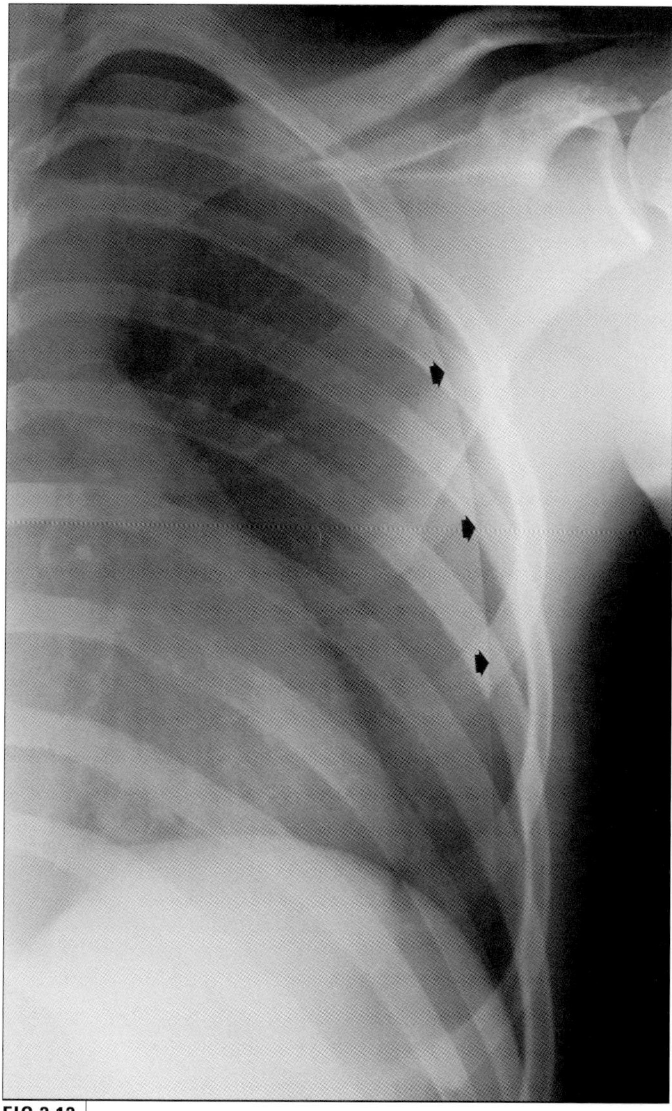

FIG 3.13

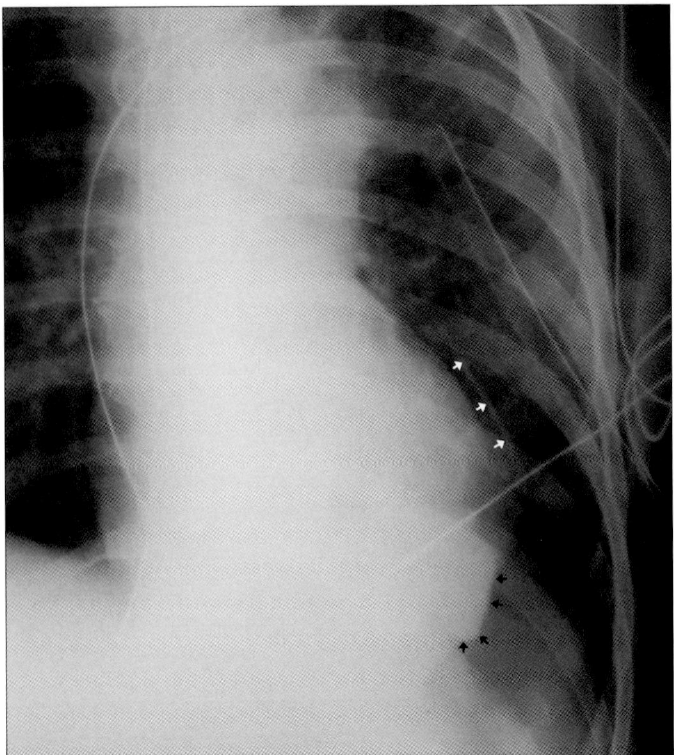

Fig. 3.14 Basal supine pneumothorax: AP view

Despite the presence of a chest tube, a left pneumothorax is present in this supine patient. It has risen to the highest part of the hemithorax in the anterior costophrenic angle. These basal supine pneumothoraces can be difficult to identify because the visceral pleural edge may not be separated from the apex or lateral chest wall. The visceral pleural edge is separated from the left cardiac margin (white arrows). The free air sharpens the cardiac outline (black arrows).

In this case there is also a band of subcutaneous emphysema lying on the outer edges of the ribs.

(See anterior sulcus sign, deep sulcus sign and double diaphragm sign in Appendix 2.)

CONSIDERATIONS IN THE YOUNG

Broadly speaking, CXRs in infants and children are indicated when there is a need to check the airways and lung fields, and to check for any gross cardiac anomalies. Ideally, the radiograph (usually an AP view for convenience) should be taken when patients are still and during full inspiration, although an expiratory X-ray may be helpful if there is concern about a foreign body and signs of air-trapping are recognised.

In young children the lung fields are relatively small and the diaphragm high. Congenital abnormalities that can be detected include diaphragmatic hernia, lung hypoplasia and lobar emphysema. The radiographic signs of asthma are more common in children than adults and include hyperinflation and bronchial wall thickening. The mediastinum is prominent because of the thymus. The thymic shadow is relatively large in the first three years and then diminishes. The thymic shadow should not be confused with lung consolidation (see sail sign, Appendix 2).

CONSIDERATIONS IN THE ELDERLY

Age-related changes should be noted in the elderly (see Table 3.4). For example, in the spine, there is increasing thoracic kyphosis from osteoporosis; and osteophytic lipping from degenerative change. The osteoporosis, if severe, may cause vertebral wedging and compression fractures. Osteophytes can also be seen in the glenohumeral and acromioclavicular joints. Calcification is common in the costal cartilages, trachea and bronchi. Note that the aorta 'unfolds' with loss of elastic tissue, as it is fixed at the aortic valve and the diaphragm hiatus. The ascending aorta bulges the right border of the upper mediastinum and the descending aorta bulges to the left. Generalised tissue wasting occurs. The loss of lung volume is accompanied by collapse of the chest wall inwards. This increases the cardiothoracic ratio to more than 50%, even when the heart itself is smaller (see Fig. 3.15). Further, loss of peripheral lung vessels leads to increased pulmonary resistance, pulmonary hypertension and prominence of the pulmonary trunks (hila).

The apical pleural cap is the thickening of the apical pleura which is a normal process of ageing. It needs to be distinguished from a Pancoast tumour (superior sulcus tumour) and from fibrosis (tuberculosis or radiation).

TABLE 3.4	Normal signs of advanced age
• Calcified costal cartilages	
• Calcified trachea and main bronchi	
• Degenerative spinal disc disease with disc space narrowing and osteophytes	
• Demineralisation of the thoracic spine and increased kyphosis	
• Aortic wall calcification	
• Loss of elastic tissue causing 'unfolding' of the aorta and arch branches. The ascending aorta projects further to the right than the superior vena cava (SVC) so that its convex border forms the right mediastinal outline	
• With unfolding and ectasia of the aortic arch, the trachea deviates more to the right as it descends	
• Tortuous descending aorta	
• Apical lung scarring	
• The lower flatter hemidiaphragms and the altered thoracic shape produce an appearance of 'senile emphysema'	

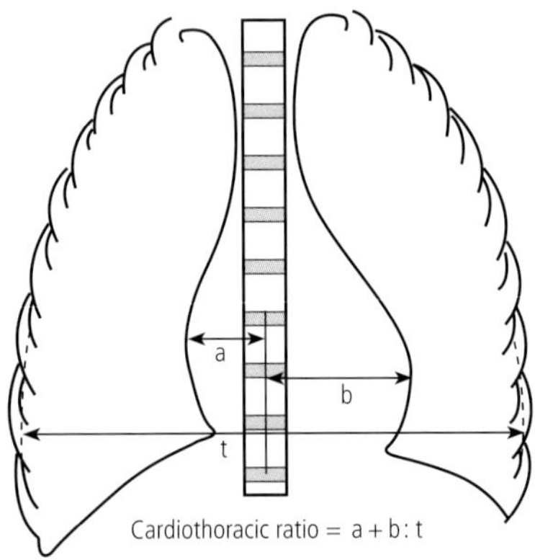

Fig. 3.15 Estimation of the cardiothoracic ratio

This estimation can only be performed on a PA film because magnification of the heart occurs on an AP film. See Figs. 1.4 and 5.3.

The most lateral aspect of the right cardiac margin is usually higher than the greatest lateral extent of the left heart border. The thoracic diameter is the widest horizontal distance between the inner margins of the ribs.

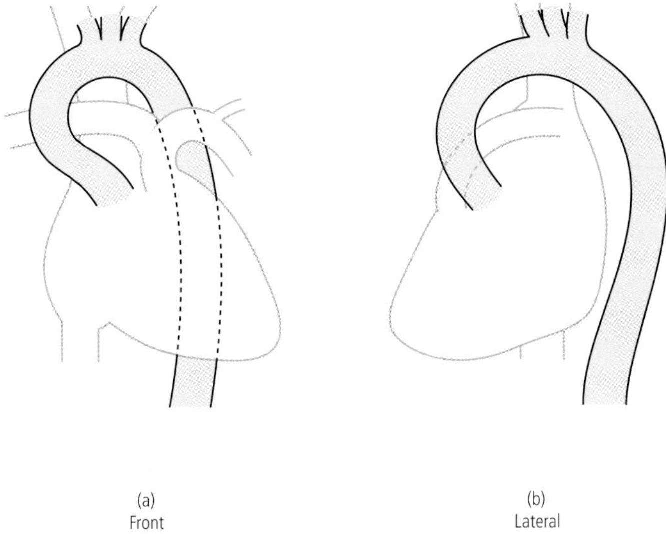

Fig. 3.16 Unfolding of the aorta: (a) frontal view; (b) lateral view
Unfolding of the aorta is due to loss of elastic tissue with aging. On the frontal view, the ascending aorta bulges to the right and the descending aorta swings more to the left. More of the descending aorta is seen on the lateral view as it is outlined by air.

LATERAL CHEST X-RAY

The purpose of the lateral view is to show another side of a three-dimensional structure (e.g. see the lungs below the diaphragmatic apices) and to help localise and diagnose abnormalities seen on the frontal film.

Usually the left lateral view is the routine. As with the PA view, this film is viewed from the 'film' side of the patient, so that for the left lateral view the film is placed with the sternum on the examiner's left; that is, it is viewed as if looking at that side of the patient. By radiographic convention, a right lateral view is performed if known pathology is on the left (see Fig. 3.7 for example). There should be a sequence of search or a mental checklist so that scrutiny is complete.

- The name and date need to be checked first so that the study corresponds to the PA view.
- Apart from satisfactory film exposure, a good technique is that the arms are elevated so that they do not hide lung detail. Check whether the ribs overlap and that there is no rotation.

- The trachea should be followed downwards from the neck to a rounded translucency—this does not correspond to the true anatomical carina. This rounded translucency represents the main bronchi.
- Check the density of the hilar shadows. Because the two hilar shadows are superimposed (combined hilar silhouette), it is difficult to distinguish the features of one from the other. However, remember that the right pulmonary artery should lie anterior to the carina with the left pulmonary artery lying above and then posterior to the carina.
- The heart shadow lies anteroinferiorly in the chest with the ascending aorta arising superiorly and joining the aortic arch. More of the descending aorta becomes visible on the lateral film as the patient ages. With the loss of the elastic tissue, the descending aorta bulges against the lung.
- If there is any exaggerated bulge of the posterior cardiac margin, consider if left atrial dilatation is present.
- Unusual densities projected over the anterior cardiophrenic angle are most likely pericardial fat pads.
- Check for any valvular or pericardial calcifications.
- Portions of lung fields need to be assessed individually. Remember that the lateral view shows superimposition of the two lungs and therefore the vascular pattern is less informative. The retrosternal and retrocardiac air spaces should have a similar 'blackness' or translucency. Reduced translucency in the retrosternal region suggests either an abnormality in the anterior mediastinum or in the anterior lungs at that level. The increasing amount of lung over the spine from above downwards should be blacker. If not, this suggests dense lung or fluid is projected over the spine (see vertebral fade-off sign, Appendix 2).
- Are the pleural fissures visible?
- The diaphragm should be examined at the same time as the lung bases. Check that the costophrenic angles are sharp and not blunted by the first signs of an effusion.
- The hemidiaphragms can be traced back posteriorly to the ribs (see big rib sign, Appendix 2). If a unilateral pleural effusion is present, only one hemidiaphragm may be visible.
- It depends on the centring whether one hemidiaphragm is projected higher than the other. If the gastric air bubble is visible, the left hemidiaphragm should lie just above it. The hemidiaphragms may be flattened in chronic airways limitation (CAL).
- Check the retrotracheal triangle (Raider's triangle). This should be a clear space between the posterior tracheal wall and the anterior margin of the thoracic spine. Increased opacity in this region could

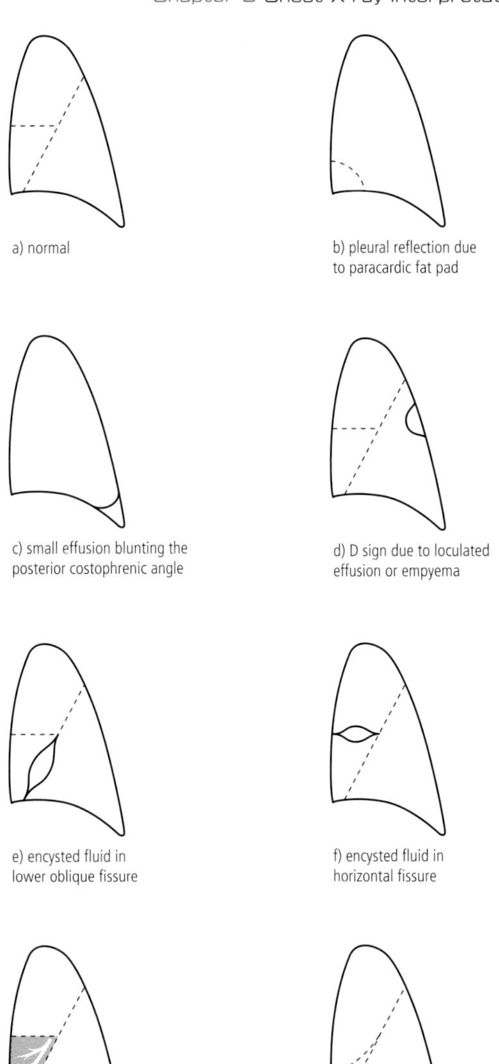

Fig. 3.17 Lateral CXR figures

be due to a mediastinal tumour or an aberrant subclavian artery. It can also be opacified by a lung tumour or consolidation projected over it.

- As with the PA film, check the soft tissues and bones. The thoracic spine and discs should be well visualised. Interoretation of the upper aspects is difficult because of the shoulders and arms; take care that the scapulae are not mistaken for lung opacities.

Another method of lateral CXR search is the ABC system—A for airways, B for bones, C for cardiac, D for diaphragm, E for effusions, F for fissures, G for gastric gas, H for hila.

LIMITATIONS OF CHEST RADIOGRAPHY

Even on a technically excellent CXR, parts of the lungs are hidden by the bones, mediastinum or diaphragm, The medial aspects of the upper zones, where there are overlapping clavicles and ribs, are particularly dangerous areas ('lawyer zones') for missing cancers.

Chest X-rays can be normal in *pulmonary embolism without infarction*. If the patient is dyspnoeic and the chest radiograph is normal, always raise the possibility of pulmonary embolism in the report. Figley et al. have said 'The principal evidence of embolism on the chest roentgenogram is often the paucity of abnormalities for a patient in such dire straits.' However, a CXR is necessary to exclude other causes for symptoms of chest pain, dyspnoea or haemoptysis.

In *asthma*, the CXR may be normal or show hyperinflation, but the degree of hyperinflation correlates poorly with the severity and reversibility of the asthma attack. In *emphysema*, the CXR can show gross morphological change such as bullae, increased lung translucency and flattened hemidiaphragms, but these signs are not always present and physiological information must be gained from lung function tests and blood gas analyses. *Inflammatory changes of the bronchi* are not visible unless they produce secondary changes in the lungs or if they cause bronchial wall thickening. Hence, *bronchiectasis* is seen only when the changes have become marked. *Dry pleurisy* and even *small effusions* are not visible. The lateral costophrenic angles will not become blunted on a frontal or PA radiograph until 100 mL of pleural fluid has collected—the first place an effusion becomes visible is at the posterior costophrenic angles on the lateral X-ray, where 50 mL of pleural fluid needs to accumulate before it becomes visible.

Similarly, *myocardial infarction* and other acute coronary syndromes show no specific radiographic signs, and the purpose of the CXR is to determine the degree of pulmonary oedema and exclude other causes of chest pain.

Moderate mediastinal lymph node enlargement and other *mediastinal abnormalities* can be hidden in the uniform mediastinal density unless there is an alteration in the mediastinal contour.

The diagnostic information obtained from AP films, either erect or supine, is less than from PA films. AP films are technically more difficult for the radiographer, leading to poor patient positioning and centring, with longer exposure times required. Fine detail of the lungs and the amount of lung visualised are reduced and cardiac size cannot be assessed. Upper lobe blood diversion cannot be ascertained on supine films. These AP films are often performed for bedridden patients to check line and tube placement, pneumothorax, lung collapse, lung consolidation and so on.

Tables 3.5 and 3.6 show structures that mimic chest abnormalities on CXR and computed tomography (CT).

TABLE 3.5 Chest X-ray mimics

Mimicked pathology	Structure
Pneumothorax	Skin fold, rib companion shadow, apical bulla, monitoring line
Pulmonary nodule	Skin mole, nipple, electrocardiogram pad, pleural plaque, sclerotic bone lesion (e g. bone island), healing rib fracture, spinal osteophyte
Apical mass/opacity	Hair locks, first rib costochondral calcification
Paratracheal mass	Ectatic innominate vessels, azygos lobe
Azygos node	Enlarged azygos vein in supine position.
Lung tumour/pneumonia	Breast prosthesis, scapula, rib fusion, pseudotumour
Right upper lobe consolidation	Infant thymus (sail sign)
Middle lobe collapse	Pectus excavatum
Lung cavity	Loculated hydropneumothorax, ulcerating breast carcinoma

(Continued)

TABLE 3.5 Chest X-ray mimics (Continued)

Mimicked pathology	Structure
Mediastinal mass	Pericardial fat pad, unfolded innominate artery, right-sided aortic arch, double aortic arch, aortic coarctation, aortic pseudocoarctation, large vertebral osteophyte, consolidated azygos lobe
Cardiomegaly	Pectus excavatum, large cardiophrenic fat pads, pericardial effusion, poor inspiration, AP view
Diaphragmatic mass	Diaphragmatic eventration
Raised hemidiaphragm	Subpulmonary effusion
Subcutaneous emphysema	Long hair braids
Pleural thickening	Extrapleural fat in an obese patient
Pneumoperitoneum	Interposition of colon above the liver (Chilaiditi syndrome)

TABLE 3.6 Computed tomography mimics

Mimicked pathology	Structure
Pulmonary embolus	Right hilar lymphatic sump of Borrie
Aortic dissection	Superior pericardial recess
Lymphadenopathy	Superior pericardial recess, aortopulmonary window

CHAPTER 4

COMMON LUNG PATHOLOGIES

The common lung pathologies are:

- pneumonia, including tuberculosis (TB) infection
- aspiration syndromes
- pulmonary oedema (see Chapter 5)
- pulmonary embolism (see Chapter 5)
- tumour
- collapse
- haemorrhage
- COPD, e.g. emphysema
- occupational lung disease
- chronic diffuse infiltrative lung disease

PNEUMONIA

Pulmonary infections can be divided into infections involving the central airways (tracheobronchitis), the small airways (bronchiolitis) and the pulmonary parenchyma (pneumonia).

Pneumonia means inflammation of the lungs. It is visualised on the radiograph as either alveolar or interstitial shadowing. Alveolar shadowing or airspace filling shows as consolidation, in this case due to an exudate. The signs of consolidation are the increased density itself, the 'air bronchogram' sign (see Appendix 2) and the 'silhouette' sign (see Appendix 2). Interstitial shadowing is characteristic of viral and *Pneumocystis jirovecii* pneumonias and shows as increased interstitial markings.

Primary pneumonia occurs in an otherwise normal lung, whereas secondary pneumonia occurs beyond bronchial occlusion, from aspiration, or in a pre-existing abnormality. The bronchial obstruction could be due to a bronchial tumour or inhaled foreign body. Aspiration may be from oropharyngeal or gastric contents, sinusitis or extrogenous fluid.

The three major aspiration syndromes are bacterial pneumonia, chemical pneumonitis and obstructive atelectasis. The aspiration of oropharyngeal flora leads to pneumonia in the gravity-dependent portions of the lungs. Aspiration of gastric juice (Mendelson syndrome) results in acute lung injury, manifesting radiographically as 'non-cardiogenic pulmonary oedema'. Aspiration of large particles can lead to obstructive atelectasis.

Acute pulmonary infection may be caused by a variety of organisms. Bacterial, mycobacterial, fungal, viral and parasitic pneumonias can all produce focal or diffuse airspace opacities on chest radiography or an interstitial pattern.

The six main radiological patterns of pneumonia are:

1. Bronchopneumonia
2. Lobar pneumonia
3. Rounded pneumonia
4. Interstitial pattern
5. Cavitatory pneumonia
6. Miliary pneumonia

1. *Bronchopneumonia*: This starts in the airways and spreads to the peribronchial alveoli with multifocal areas of consolidation. These patchy, inhomogeneous shadows can coalesce. The bronchopneumonia pattern is commonly observed with staphylococcal infection.
2. *Lobar pneumonia*: In this case, the inflammatory changes are confined to a lobe (see Fig. 4.1) or can be multilobar. Classically, it occurs with *Streptococcus pneumoniae* (pneumococcus) but also with *Klebsiella*, primary TB and *Staphylococcus*. *Klebsiella* pneumonia can produce the bulging fissure sign (see Appendix 2) due to the associated oedema.

   The lobar pattern of consolidation usually begins as a peripheral opacity. The resultant confluent, homogeneous consolidation often has air bronchograms present. The infection spreads through the lung via small channels—the canals of Lambert and the pores of Kohn—rather than the bronchioles. It therefore crosses pulmonary segments but is limited by pleural boundaries.

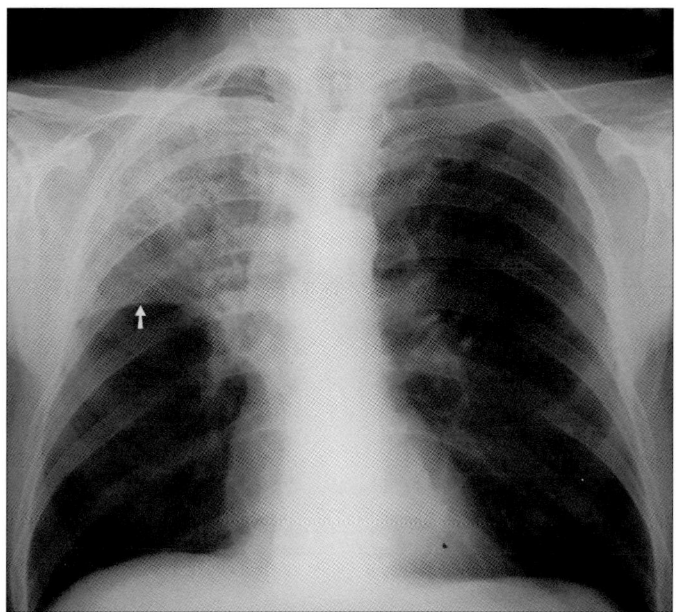

FIG 4.1a

Fig. 4.1 Right upper lobe consolidation: (a) PA view; (b) lateral view. Increased opacity is seen in the shape of the right upper lobe. The slight elevation of the horizontal fissure indicates that a degree of collapse is also present. This slight collapse would explain the rightward deviation of the trachea.

If this consolidation was denser, the air bronchogram sign (see Appendix 2) might be visible with more loss of the mediastinal silhouette.

The commonest cause of a lobar pneumonia is *Streptococcus pneumoniae*.

If the consolidation fails to clear, an endobronchial mass causing a post-obstructive pneumonia needs to be considered (see differential diagnosis of lobar pneumonia, Appendix 3).

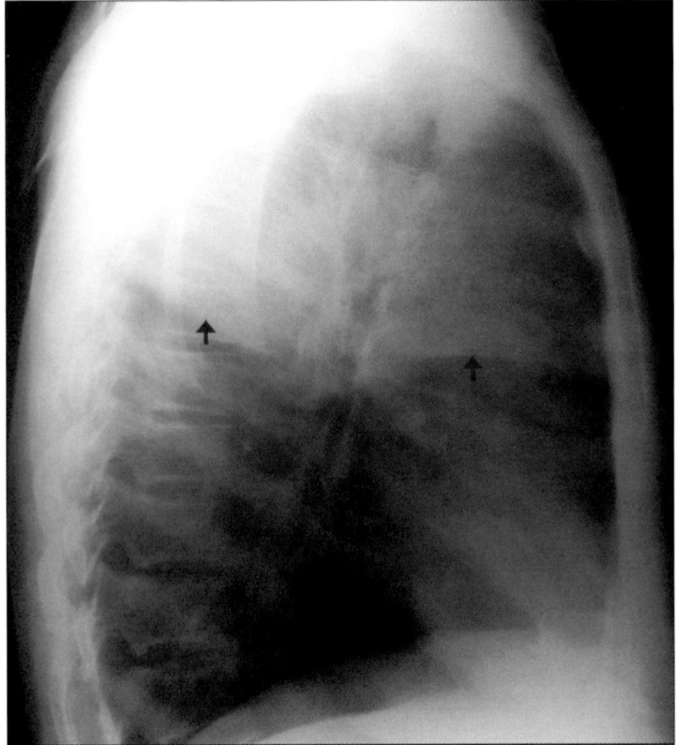

FIG 4.1b

Fig. 4.1 Right upper lobe consolidation: (a) PA view; (b) lateral view.

3. *Rounded pneumonia*: This can occur with staphylococcal infection in children and in fungal infection (e.g. aspergilloma and toruloma). Occasionally, pneumococcal pneumonia appears as a focal nodule or mass like and is called 'round pneumonia'.
4. *Interstitial pattern*: This occurs with viral pneumonias and *Pneumocystis jirovecii* and occasionally with *Mycoplasma* infections.
5. *Cavitatory pneumonia*: This implies that necrosis has occurred with drainage into the bronchial tree. Acute cavitation is seen with *Staphylococcus* and anaerobic bacteria. Chronic cavitation occurs with TB, histoplasmosis and coccidiomycosis (see Fig. 4.2 on page 74).
6. *Miliary pneumonia* (see Fig. 4.3 on pages 75–76).

Another classification of pneumonia is based on the clinical situation in which the infection occurs:

- community-acquired pneumonia
- nosocomial pneumonia (hospital-acquired)
- aspiration pneumonia
- pneumonia in the immunocompromised host.

Streptococcal, mycoplasmal and viral pneumonias are the commonest community-acquired pneumonias in adults. Hospital-acquired pneumonia is usually due to gram-negative bacilli, staphylococci, anaerobic organisms and *Streptococcus pneumoniae*.

The predisposing factors for nosocomial infection are elderly age, decreased mentation, ICU admission, endotracheal intubation, recent thoracic or upper abdominal surgery.

Types of pneumonia

- In nearly half the patients, the aetiological agent is not identified.
- Community-acquired pneumonia is the most common cause of acute lung infection in immunocompromised and immunocompetent patients.
- Streptococcal pneumonia is the commonest cause of bacterial pneumonia. The classic manifestation is a lobar pneumonia.
- Staphylococcal pneumonia is the most frequent cause of bronchopneumonia and is the usual secondary invader after viral influenza infection. It is an important cause of nosocomial infections and is a complication of infected intravenous catheters.
- Atypical pneumonia is a subset of pneumonias which do not have the typical symptoms. The patients have a non-productive cough and extrapulmonary manifestations, such as headache, myalgia and diarrhoea. Included as causes in this group of pneumonias are *Mycoplasma, Legionella* and *Chlamydia*. More recently the severe acute respiratory syndrome (SARS) coronavirus has caused epidemics of atypical pneumonia.
- *Mycoplasma* pneumonia usually shows as a diffuse interstitial fine reticulonodular pattern or patchy consolidation.
- Legionnaires' disease (*Legionella* pneumonia) is usually a cause of local epidemics from infected air-conditioning systems.
- Respiratory syncytial virus (RSV) is the most common viral pneumonia in children whereas influenza is the most common in adults. Viral pneumonia can be particularly severe in elderly and immunocompromised patients. They may have a dry hacking cough with minimal radiographic findings. H5NI is a new and unusually virulent strain of avian influenza A. The main viruses

causing viral pneumonia in immunocompromised patients are cytomegalovirus, varicella zoster and herpes.

- *Pneumocystis jirovecii* pneumonia is a complicating illness in acquired immunodeficiency syndrome (AIDS) or immunosuppressed patients, including transplant patients and those on long-term steroid therapy. *Pneumocystis* is named from its cystic structure rather than the pneumatocoeles it can produce. The usual presentation shows a chest radiograph with fine symmetrical reticular opacification.
- SARS is caused by a coronavirus. The chest radiograph may show ground-glass opacity or consolidation. If the CXR is normal, then high-resolution computed tomography (HRCT) is necessary. Cavitation, calcification, lymphadenopathy and pleural effusion are not features of this disease.
- Inhalational anthrax causes a haemorrhagic pneumonia with hilar and mediastinal lymphadenopathy.
- Crytogenic-organising pneumonia is a chronic focal process of consolidation that is treated with steroids.
- Chronic eosinophilic pneumonia produces the symptoms of dyspnoea, fever, chills, night sweats and weight loss. Blood eosinophilia, peripheral consolidation and dramatic response to corticosteroid treatment are the hallmarks of diagnosis, as is the 'reverse butterfly' appearance on CXR.
- Lipoid pneumonia occurs usually in elderly patients and results from oil aspiration. It is not an infective pneumonia.
- Aspergillus can cause a spectrum of diseases dependent on the patient's immune and pulmonary status: non-invasive aspergillosis (mycetoma), semi-invasive aspergillosis, invasive aspergillosis, allergic bronchopulmonary aspergillosis and allergic bronchitis (see Figs. 4.6 and 4.9).
- Toruloma is a mass-like infection of the fungus *Cryptococcus neoformans*. It can mimic a lung carcinoma.
- Histoplasma, Blastomyces and Coccidioides are regionally endemic fungi in the USA and cause community-acquired pneumonia in healthy adults and immunosuppressed patients.
- Multilobar bacterial pneumonia has increased morbidity and mortality compared to unilobar pneumonia.
- Bacterial pneumonia is the commonest cause for consolidation in adults. Bacterial pneumonia typically presents as an acute illness with chest pain, chills, high fever and cough production of purulent sputum.

  Parapneumonic pleural effusions are a common finding with bacterial infections.

- Hydrocarbon pneumonia follows aspiration of kerosene or other hydrocarbons. It produces pulmonary oedema and lower zone opacities.
- Most cases of organising pneumonia are idiopathic, i.e. cryptogenic organising pneumonia. Patients with COP typically present with a several-month history of non-productive cough, low-grade fever, malaise and shortness of breath. COP responds well to steroids.
- Chickenpox (Varicella) pneumonia show multiple lung nodules which later calcify unlike miliary TB which does not calcify. These calcified scars are 3 mm wide.
- The air-space filling in the bronchoalveolar carcinoma can mimic infective consolidation.

TUBERCULOSIS

Tuberculosis is due to infection by *Mycobacterium tuberculosis*, usually in the respiratory tract.

Primary TB is usually asymptomatic, with inhalation of airborne droplets causing a focal area of consolidation with lymphadenopathy in the hilum. Lymphadenopathy may also be present in the contiguous nodes. The combination of the focal pulmonary lesion (Ghon lesion) and the lymphadenopathy is the primary Rathke complex. The enlarged lymph nodes can cause bronchial compression and obstructive atelectasis. The Ghon lesion usually heals into a focus of calcification but can persist as a tuberculoma.

A number of factors can predispose to reactivation, including malnutrition, diabetes mellitus, alcoholism, ageing, drug-induced immunosuppression, disease-induced immunosuppression and AIDS. This post-primary or reactivation TB is common in the apical and posterior segments of the upper lobes and the apical segments of the lower lobes. These segments are characterised by a high ventilation/perfusion (V/Q) ratio and relatively high Po_2 levels. A chronic patchy area of consolidation with cavitation occurs (see Fig. 4.2). Hilar and mediastinal lymphadenopathy are not a feature in immunocompetent patients.

Other patterns of reactivation include lobar pneumonia, diffuse bronchopneumonia, endobronchial TB and tuberculous pleuritis. Miliary TB is due to haematogenous dissemination and can complicate both primary and reactivation disease (see Fig. 4.3).

The healing of the pulmonary lesions is manifest by reduction in the area of consolidation, decrease in cavity size, fibrosis and calcification.

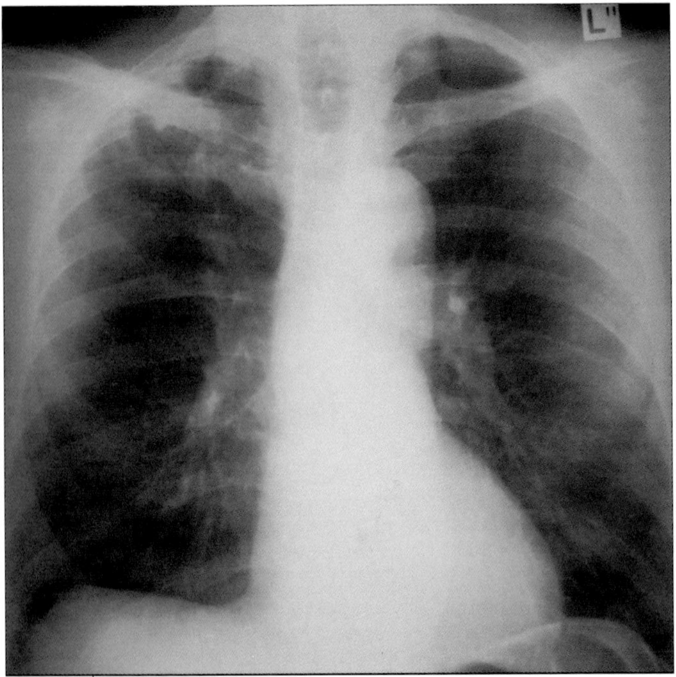

FIG 4.2a

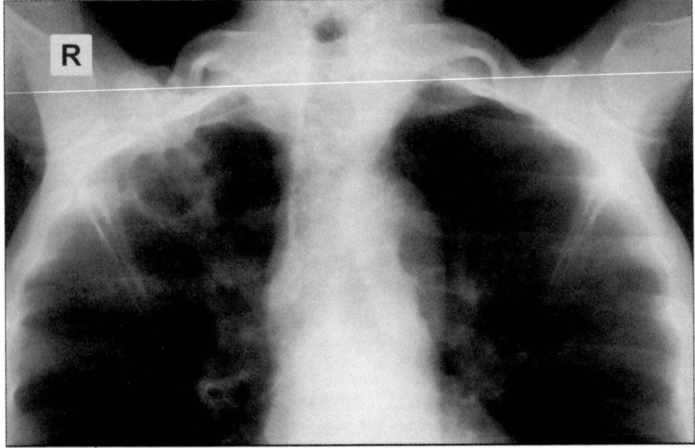

FIG 4.2b

Fig. 4.2 Tuberculous cavity: (a) PA view; (b) lordotic view

There is a cavitating lung lesion in the right upper lobe which is partially hidden by the overlying bones on the standard PA view. The lordotic view provides a better demonstration (see differential diagnosis of cavitating lung lesion, Appendix 3).

Fig. 4.3 Miliary tuberculosis: (a) PA view; (b) magnified view

The widespread multiple 1–2 mm nodules are so-called because of their resemblance of millet seeds. They are uniform in size and distribution. Massive haematogenous spread results in multiple mycobacterial foci caught in capillary sieves of the interstitium. This miliary disease may take up to six weeks to become apparent on chest radiographs, although CT may allow earlier detection of very small nodules.

Miliary tuberculosis usually occurs as a progression of primary tuberculosis but can also be a serious complication of reactivation tuberculosis. Miliary TB does not leave residual calcifications (see differential diagnosis of miliary nodules, Appendix 3).

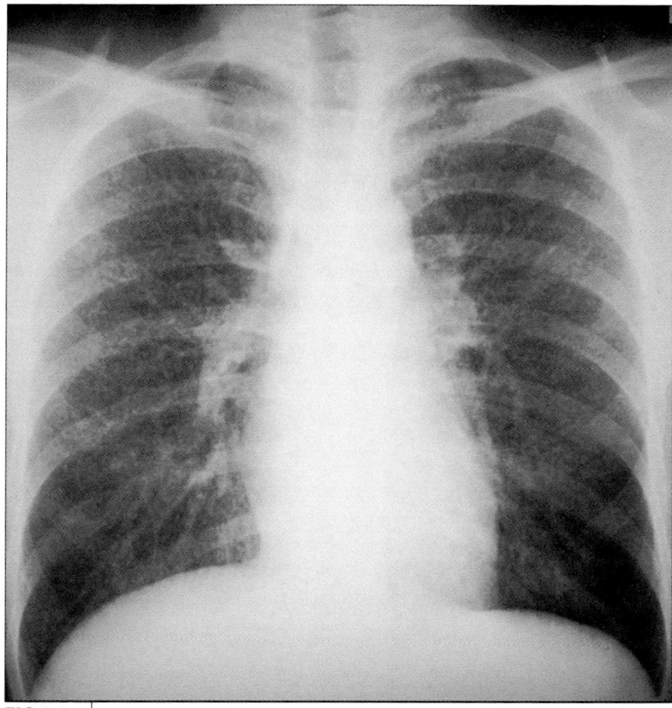

FIG 4.3a

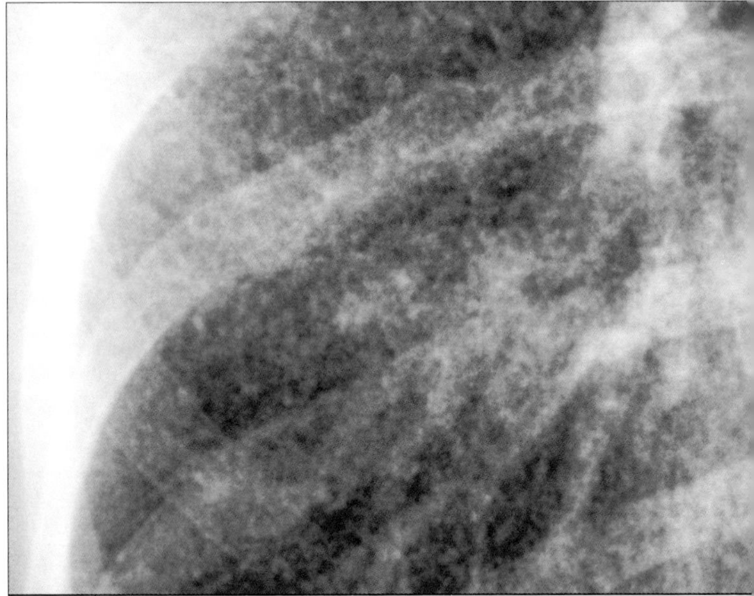

FIG 4.3b

Fig. 4.3 Miliary tuberculosis: (a) PA view; (b) magnified view

Pulmonary complications include bronchiectasis, pneumothorax, bronchopleural fistula, bronchial stenosis and broncholiths. Pleural complications are empyema and calcific fibrothorax (see Fig. 4.4). The TB may extend to extrathoracic sites, such as the intestine, kidneys, spine and central nervous system.

The type of pulmonary TB in AIDS patients depends on the patient's CD4 lymphocyte count. If the CD4 count is below 200/µL, the pattern resembles primary TB, but if it is above 200/µL, it is more like reactivation TB.

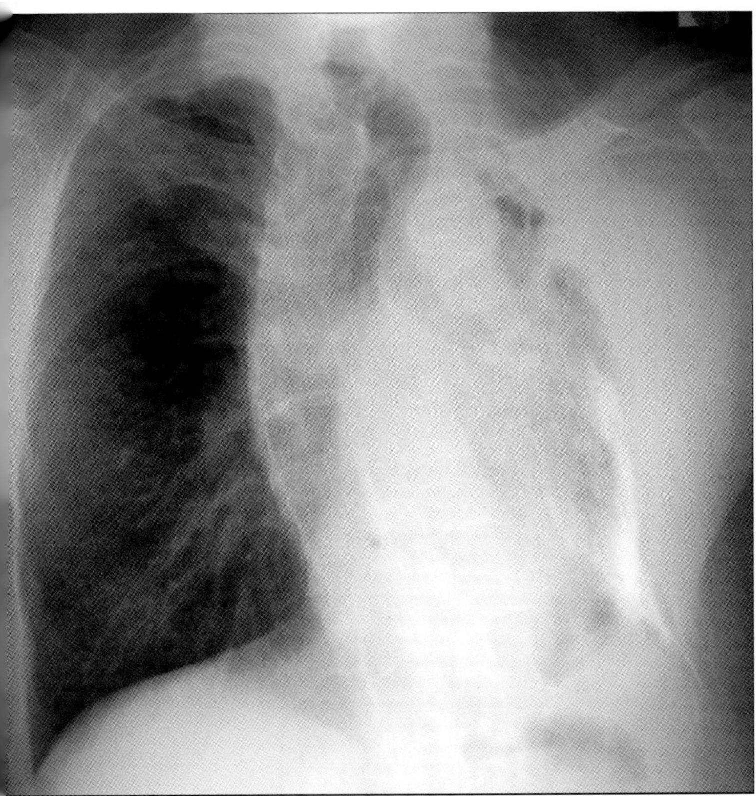

Fig. 4.4 Tuberculous calcific fibrothorax: PA view

There is gross destruction of the left lung by previous TB producing marked fibrosis. The fibrosis has shrunk the lung and caused mediastinal shift. This presumably has occurred before adult life, with a developmental scoliosis and small left hemithorax. Only a small amount of aerated left lung is present. Follow-up films or comparison with earlier films would be necessary to exclude on-going disease.

Marked generalised pleural thickening is present with pleural calcification seen over the lower zone.

The right lung shows pleural thickening and scarring at the apex; a calcified focus is seen in the right mid-zone.

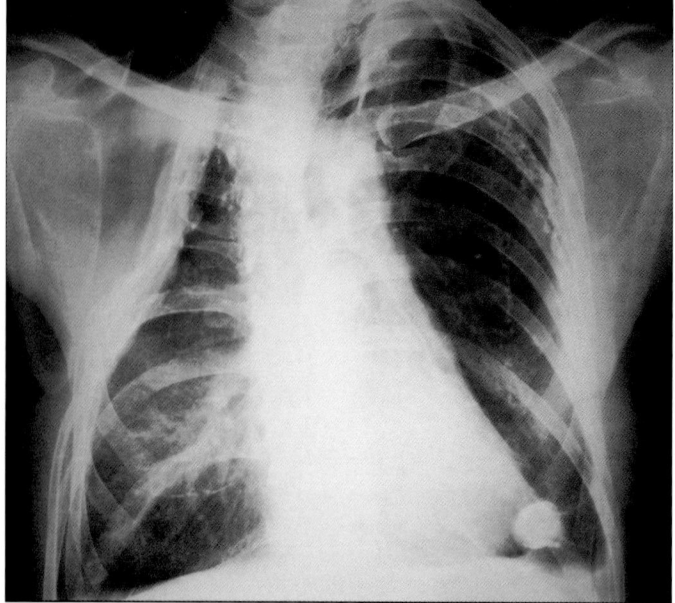

Fig. 4.5 Right thoracoplasty

Thoracoplasty was a previously performed surgical procedure where the chest wall was collapsed inwards to collapse TB-infected cavitated lung in the pre-antibiotic era.

There is evidence of previous left pleural tuberculosis with pleural calcifications. In addition, there is a prominent calcified granuloma in the left lung base.

Over the right upper zone there is evidence of a thoracoplasty.

Fig 4.6 Pulmonary mycetomas

The upper zones are scarred and cavitated from tuberculosis infection or possibly semi-invasive aspergillus itself. Within each upper zone cavity, a rounded mycetoma (aspergilloma) is visible. The fungus ball consists of aspergillus hyphae, mucus and cellular debris.

The right mid-zone consolidation is highly suggestive that semi-invasive aspergillus infection is also present.

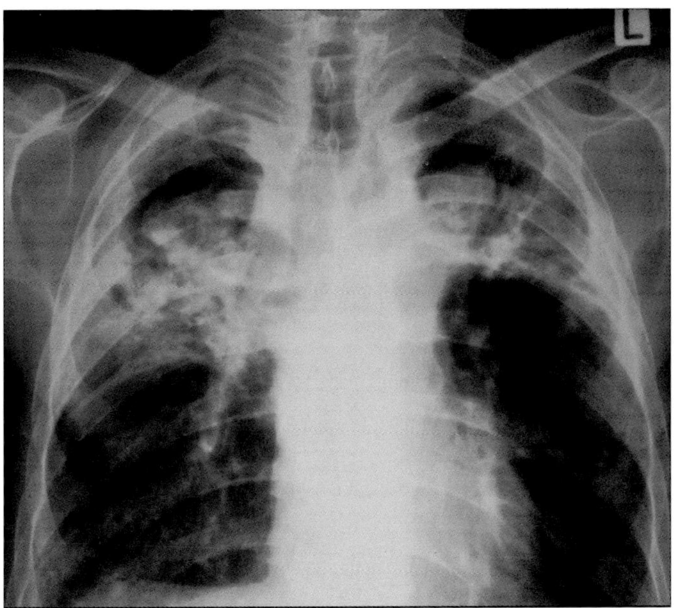

FIG 4.6

4

ASPIRATION SYNDROMES

Aspiration describes the intake of solid or liquid materials into the airways and lungs. With the patient in a supine position, the posterior segment of the upper lobes and the superior segment of the lower lobes are the most commonly involved.

The major aspiration syndromes are:

1. bacterial pneumonia
2. chemical pneumonitis
3. exogenous lipid pneumonia
4. obstructive atelectasis
5. near drowning
6. meconium aspiration syndrome.

The aspiration of oropharyngeal flora (mixed anaerobes) leads to pneumonia. On a microscopic level, inhalation of infected aerosols is the mechanism of acquiring community and nosocomial pneumonias.

Aspiration of gastric juice (Mendelson syndrome) results in acute lung injury manifesting radiographically as 'non-cardiogenic pulmonary oedema'. A similar chemical pneumonitis can occur following aspiration of hyperosmolar contrast media, e.g. Gastrografin. Although inert, barium sulphate aspiration as a complication of a barium swallow study can cause an acute inflammatory pneumonitis.

Repeated aspiration or inhalation of mineral oil or vegetable oil causes a chronic exogenous lipoid pneumonia. Common causes are bedtime oral intake of mineral oil for constipation or the frequent use of oily nose drops for chronic rhinitis. This is different from the acute exogenous lipoid pneumonia (fire-eater pneumonia) that can be caused by aspirating liquid paraffin (kerosene) and petroleum.

Aspiration of large particles including food particles and teeth can lead to obstructive atelectasis.

In near drowning, it is the volume of water aspirated that is more significant than if it is fresh water or salt water. Pulmonary oedema is the result of a massive aspiration and can be complicated by pneumonia if the water is contaminated.

Meconium aspiration syndrome is a serious condition in which the distressed fetus or newborn breathes in faeces and amniotic fluid before or during delivery causing chemical pneumonitits (see Chapter 10).

TUMOUR

Thoracic neoplasms can occur in the airways, lungs, mediastinum, pleura or chest wall.

A solitary pulmonary nodule is a well-circumscribed parenchymal mass 3 cm or less in diameter (see Fig. 4.7). There are a number of different diagnostic possibilities (see list of differential diagnoses, Appendix 3). If calcification is present within the nodule, it is most likely either a tuberculous granuloma or a hamartoma. Calcification is a good sign to exclude malignancy. Further work-up with CT scanning is required to see if it contains fat or if it has appearances suggesting infarction or pneumonia. Other forms of work-up include CT densitometry, serial CT scans with volumetric analysis and positron emission tomography (PET) with fluorodeoxyglucose (FDG). If the nodule cannot be proven to be benign, it must be biopsied or excised.

Malignant lung tumours are divided histologically and simply into small cell and non-small cell carcinomas. Small cell carcinoma

Fig. 4.7 Middle lobe tumour: (a) PA view; (b) lateral view; (c) CT scan

There is a 3.5 cm tumour in the anterior aspect of the medial segment of the middle lobe. It is clearly separated from the right heart border and not involved in any lung collapse. Vessels from the inferior part of the hilum are visible through the mass. (See hilum overlay sign, Appendix 2.)

Justifiable questions to ask from the film are:

- Is the patient a smoker?
- Is there history or symptoms of any extrapulmonary primary tumour and are any previous films available for comparison?

Because there is a strong possibility that this is a malignant mass, signs of metastatic disease, such as hilar and mediastinal lymphadenopathy, pleural effusion or other lung nodules, need to be recognised. (See differential diagnosis of solitary pulmonary nodule, Appendix 3.) Note that the term 'coin lesion' is best avoided. Although it describes the shadow cast, it does not describe the three-dimensional structure.

Critical issues:

- If this is an isolated bronchogenic carcinoma (T2 N0 M0) and is surgically resected, the five-year survival is about 50%.
- If this is a solitary metastatic deposit, the common primary sources are likely to be colon, breast, renal, melanoma or testicular. The chance of a metastasis is very low if there is no history or symptoms of a primary tumour.
- The Fleischner Society recommends using the word 'nodule' for a lesion up to 3 cm in diameter and a 'mass' for a lesion greater than 3 cm in diameter. This distinction is not rigid for other authorities.

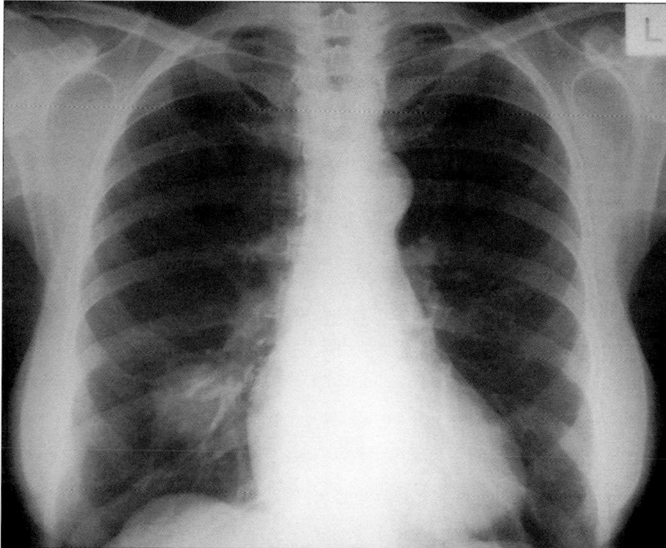

FIG 4.7a

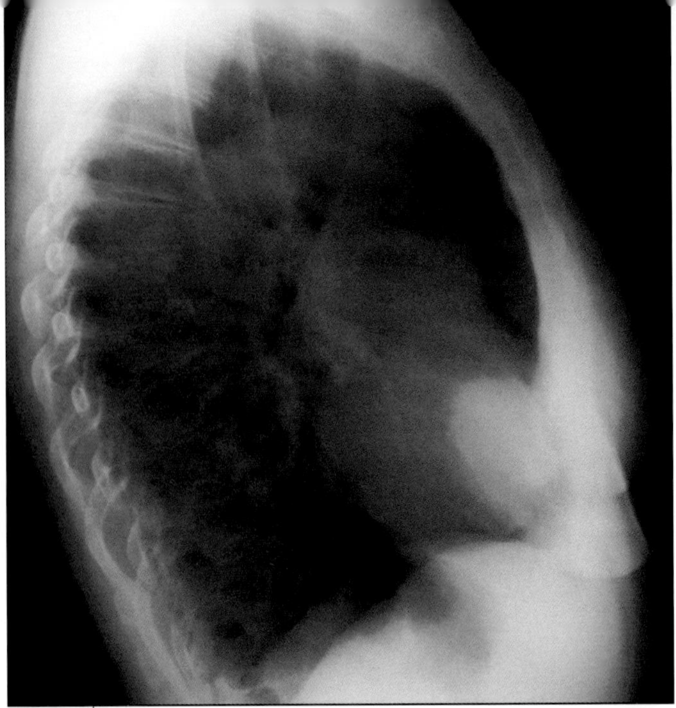

FIG 4.7b

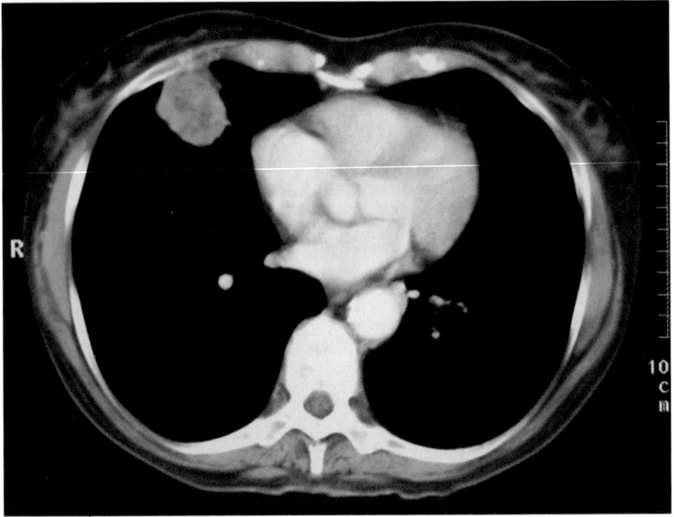

FIG 4.7c

accounts for 20% of lung cancers and is its most aggressive type with two-thirds of patients having metastases at presentation.

Ideally, surgical resection is the best treatment of limited primary tumours. Therefore, the tumour–node–metastasis (TNM) staging system is used to facilitate decision making.

The TNM staging is a system of grading of the primary tumour, regional lymph nodes and distant metastases. The International Staging System for non-small cell carcinoma further grades the tumour in terms of prognosis.

The critical division is between stages IIIA and IIIB: stage IIIA is extensive but resectable disease whereas stage IIIB is irresectable disease.

Besides active and passive tobacco smoking, occupational and other environmental factors may be responsible for the development of lung carcinoma. Asbestos exposure increases the risk of developing lung cancer by at least 5 times compared to non-smokers. In addition, there is a synergistic effect between smoking and asbestos exposure. The accentuated risk is up to 100 times that of the non-smoking non-exposed population.

Asbestos exposure also increases the risk of developing mesothelioma but there is a latency period of 20–40 years. Unlike lung carcinoma, cigarette smoking is not an aetiological factor in mesothelioma.

Even though chest radiography and CT scanning provide important information, other tests, such as bronchoscopy, PET scanning and mediastinoscopy, are useful in preoperative evaluation. However, the actual findings at thoracotomy will influence the surgeon's decision making.

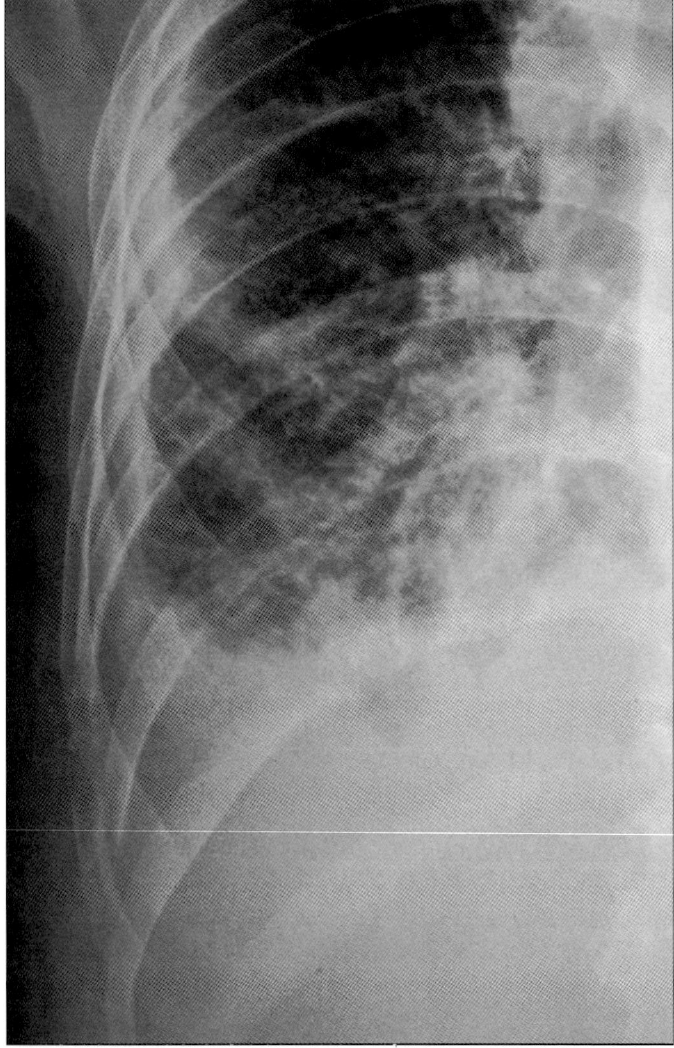

Fig. 4.8 Lymphangitic carcinomatosis

The increased pulmonary interstitial shadowing is due to 'lymphangitis carcinomatosa'. Kerley B lines due to lymphatic infiltration and obstruction are evident, simulating interstitial oedema. The clue is the masses at the right hilum. Besides the pleural effusion, there are erosions of the lateral aspects of the right lower ribs.

TABLE 4.1	CXR manifestations of carcinoma
Primary lung carcinoma	
• solitary pulmonary nodule	
• large pulmonary mass	
• cavitating mass (squamous cell carcinoma)	
• hilar mass/lymphadenopathy	
• mediastinal widening	
• lobar or segmental collapse (endobronchial lesion)	
• GGO (alveolar cell carcinoma)	
• 'persisting pneumonia'	
• scar carcinoma (+/– calcium)	
• asymmetrical apical pleural 'thickening' (Pancoast tumour, Superior Sulcus tumour)	
• carcinomatous lymphangitis	
Metastatic disease	
• pulmonary nodules (solitary, multiple, miliary)	
• hilar and/or mediastinal lymphadenopathy	
• lymphangitis carcinomatosis	
• lung collapse (endobronchial deposits)	
• pleural effusions	
• bony metastases	

DIFFUSE PULMONARY HAEMORRHAGE

Diffuse pulmonary haemorrhage occurs when there is widespread haemorrhage from the lung microvasculature into the alveolar spaces. It can occur with conditions associated with glomerulonephritis, immune complex and antiglomerular basement membrane disease. Goodpasture syndrome has pulmonary haemorrhage associated with glomerulonephritis and antiglomerular basement antibodies. Alternatively, idiopathic pulmonary haemosiderosis (IPH) is a disorder without immunological associations or renal disease. The aetiology of IPH is unknown and it eventually leads to lung fibrosis.

The typical findings are haemoptysis and anaemia with the chest radiograph showing diffuse alveolar consolidation.

CHRONIC OBSTRUCTIVE PULMONARY DISEASE

Chronic obstructive pulmonary disease is an umbrella term for a group of diseases that cause chronic or recurrent obstruction to airflow. These are:

1. asthma
2. bronchiectasis
3. chronic bronchitis/bronchiolitis
4. emphysema
5. cystic fibrosis.

With the exception of cystic fibrosis, the four principal disorders may coexist in various degrees in the same patient.

Chronic bronchitis has the clinical diagnosis of the presence of chronic productive cough for three months in each of two successive years where other causes have been excluded. Emphysema, however, has the pathological diagnosis of abnormal, permanent enlargement of the air spaces distal to the terminal bronchiole, accompanied by destruction of their walls (but without obvious fibrosis).

Asthma

The diagnosis of asthma is based on the clinical history and findings as well as the physiological tests showing reversible airflow obstruction. Also there is airway inflammation and hyper-reactivity of the airways to a variety of stimuli. At least two-thirds have atopic asthma—immediate type 1 hypersensitivity reaction to a specific antigen or allergen.

An obstructive neoplasm, inhaled foreign body, congestive heart failure ('cardiac asthma') and bronchiectasis can also produce wheezing and are clinical mimics of asthma.

A chest radiograph is indicated on initial work-up to exclude these other causes of wheezing, when the acute attack is severe enough for admission to hospital, or when complications are suspected. These complications include pneumothorax, pneumomediastinum or pneumonia.

In uncomplicated asthma, the chest radiograph may be normal. Although there is an increase in the residual lung volume and the total lung capacity, this may not be enough to cause flattening of the hemidiaphragms and other signs of hyperinflation.

In chronic asthma, bronchial wall thickening, areas of atelectasis (due to mucous plugging) and hyperinflation may be seen on the CXR. In 2% of asthmatics there may be signs of allergic bronchopulmonary aspergillosis with mucoid impaction and central bronchiectasis (see Fig. 4.9).

Bronchiectasis

Bronchiectasis is abnormal permanent dilatation of the bronchi. These ectatic bronchi often show inflammatory wall thickening and are the result of many different diseases, both congenital and acquired. (See differential diagnosis of bronchiectasis, Appendix 3). Reid classified them into three main types: cylindrical, varicose and cystic (saccular). Cystic bronchiectasis is the most advanced type (see Fig. 4.10).

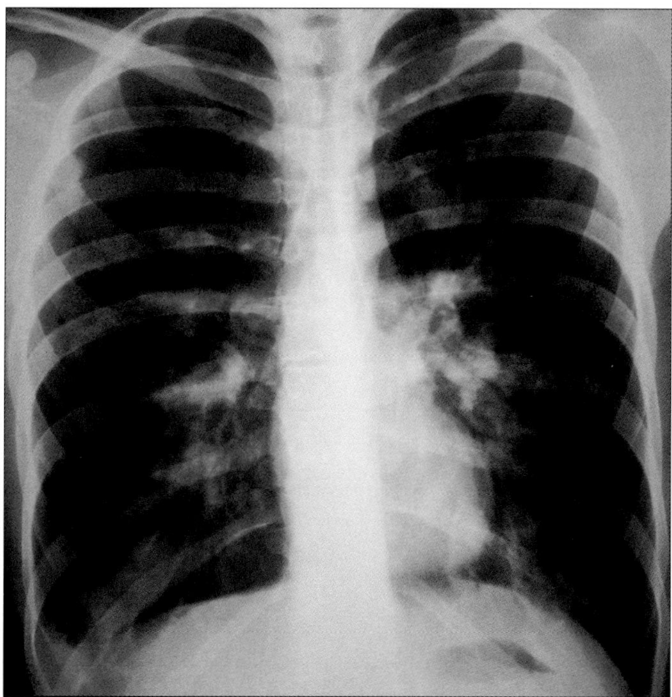

Fig. 4.9 Allergic bronchopulmonary aspergillosis

This disease occurs exclusively in asthmatics where there is a hypersensitivity reaction to aspergillus colonising the airways.

Opacities are seen in both lungs due to mucoid impaction in ectatic bronchi. Some mucous plugs are seen more centrally at the hila.

The variable obstructive pattern on lung function testing is due to the varying degree of associated obstructive bronchiolitis.

The CXR has limited reliability in showing bronchiectasis although it can demonstrate the moderate and severe forms. CT and HRCT show bronchiectasis reliably so that now bronchography is an obsolete test.

A common plain film finding in this condition is tramline shadowing representing thick-walled cylindrically dilated bronchi. Mucus-filled bronchi may show the 'gloved finger' or 'toothpaste shadow' sign. Cystic bronchiectasis will show as cystic areas; some with air fluid levels due to dependent mucus and exudate (see Fig. 4.10).

Other types of bronchiectasis are:

- central bronchiectasis occurs classically with ABPA
- wet and dry bronchiectasis refers to whether associated infection is present or not
- reversible bronchiectasis is by definition not true bronchiectasis and refers to the transient dilatation occurring after pneumonia or atelectasis
- traction bronchiectasis (CT finding) is anatomically more due to ectasia of the bronchioles which are stretched by the surrounding fibrosis.

Chronic bronchitis

In many patients with chronic bronchitis, the CXR is normal.

The important indication for the CXR in chronic bronchitis is to rule out other causes of cough and sputum expectoration. In many patients with chronic bronchitis, the CXR is normal.

The radiographic signs indicating chronic bronchitis are bronchial wall thickening and increased lung markings ('dirty lung'). These small ill-defined linear opacities are a subjective finding and have not been fully elucidated by HRCT. Associated signs of emphysema may be seen in these cigarette-smoking patients.

Emphysema

The different types of emphysema have been described according to their location in the secondary pulmonary lobule: centrilobular (centriacinar), panlobular (panacinar) and paraseptal (distal acinar).

Centriacinar emphysema is the most common form of emphysema and is due to smoking. The destruction of the alveolar walls begins in the central portion of the secondary pulmonary lobule, worse in the upper lobes. The upper lungs are the most severely affected because of the greater ventilation/perfusion ratio and also because of the slower 'wash-out' of the smoke compared to the lower lobes. The smoke particulate matter usually deposits in the second-order respiratory bronchioles.

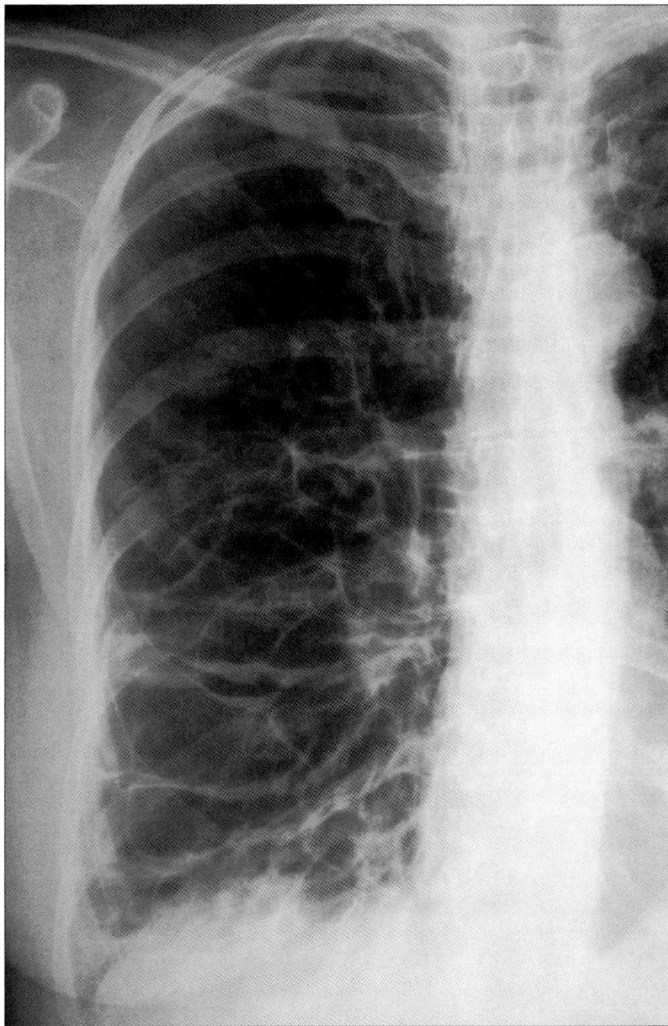

4

Fig. 4.10 Cystic bronchiectasis
Multiple cysts are seen in the right mid and lower zones due to cystic or saccular bronchiectasis. This is the most severe form of bronchiectasis.

Panlobular emphysema typically occurs in patients with alpha-1-antitrypsin deficiency and is most severe in the lower zones.

Paraseptal emphysema occurs in the distal part of the secondary pulmonary lobule and is associated with ageing. Coalescence of paraseptal emphysema leads to the formation of bullae.

The chest X-ray is insensitive for detecting mild emphysema. Moderate and severe emphysema show varying amounts of lung destruction and pulmonary hyperinflation. The signs of lung destruction are increased lung lucency, reduced vessel markings, and bullae. The signs of hyperinflation include flattening of the hemidiaphragms, increased anteroposterior chest dimension ('barrel chest'), enlargement of the retrosternal clear space, saber sheath trachea, increased lung height and the 'hanging drop' heart. When secondary pulmonary arterial hypertension develops, there is enlargement of the central pulmonary arteries and the right heart.

Emphysematous bullae are avascular air-containing cystic spaces that are more than 1 cm in diameter. The main complications of bullae are pneumothorax, infection and haemorrhage.

Bullectomy and lung volume reduction surgery are surgical options in the appropriate patients to improve lung function.

Other types of emphysema are:

- paracicatricial emphysema occurs adjacent to areas of fibrosis, for example, adjacent to progressive massive fibrosis (conglomerate masses) in patients with silicosis. The scarring stretches the adjacent lung by traction.
- combined pulmonary fibrosis and emphysema (CPFE). By strict definition, pure emphysema is not associated with fibrosis (see CPFE syndrome, Appendix 1).
- compensatory 'emphysema'. This occurs when the remaining lung expands to fill the space left by a collapsed or excised portion of lung. This is not really emphysema.
- congenital lobar emphysema is a cause of respiratory distress in infants. The hyperinflated lung can cause a shift of the mediastinum.
- pulmonary interstitial emphysema. Small areas of lucency are seen on the chest radiograph of intubated premature infant as a complication.
- unilateral emphysema. See MacLeod syndrome or Swyer–James syndrome.
- 'bong lung'. Cannabis smokers have a propensity to develop an accelerated form of emphysema with giant bullae and complicating pneumothoraces.
- mediastinal 'emphysema' is air in the mediastinum. (See causes of pneumomediastinum, Appendix 3.)
- subcutaneous emphysema is air in the subcutaneous tissue. This

can be an extension of pneumomediastinum, due to trauma, or occur with pleural catheter placement.

OCCUPATIONAL LUNG DISEASES

Inhalational and other exposures to irritants in the workplace can cause lung disease. For example, some inhaled dusts can produce fibrosis in the lungs. Table 4.2 shows a list of common occupational lung diseases.

TABLE 4.2 Occupational lung diseases
Asbestos dust inhalation
• Pleural plaques • Rounded atelectasis • Pleural effusions • Asbestosis • Mesothelioma and carcinoma
Pneumoconiosis
• Silicosis progressive massive fibrosis • Coal workers' pneumoconiosis
Interstitial fibrosis (fibrosing alveolitis)
• Paraquat poisoning • Asbestosis
Extrinsic allergic alveolitis
• Farmer's lung • Bagassosis • Humidifier fever
Bronchogenic carcinoma
• Asbestos • Nickel, uranium, cadmium • Passive smoking
Chemical pneumonitis
• Inhaled aerosols
Beryllium pneumopathy
• Acute: tracheobronchitis and pulmonary oedema • Chronic: sarcoid-like
Asthma

Pneumoconiosis ('dusty lungs') is occupational lung disease due to the lungs' reaction to inhaled dusts (see Table 4.3).

4

TABLE 4.3 Pneumonconiosis
Inorganic dusts
• without fibrosis iron, tin and barium
• with fibrosis silica, coal dust
• with chemical pneumonitis beryllium
• carcinogenic dusts radioactive dusts, asbestos, arsenic
• causing giant cell interstitial pneumonia (GIP) cobalt, tungsten carbide ('hard metal disease')
Organic dusts (extrinsic allergic alveolitis/hypersensitivity pneumonitis)
• mouldy hay – farmer's lung sugar cane dust – bagassosis
• cotton dust – byssinosis bird excreta – pigeon breeder's lung budgerigar fancier's lung

CHRONIC INFILTRATIVE DIFFUSE LUNG DISEASE

There are over 150 chronic infiltrative lung diseases, with twelve diseases accounting for 90% of cases. These diseases are:

- usual interstitial pneumonia/idiopathic pulmonary fibrosis (UIP/IPF)
- asbestosis
- desquamative interstitial pneumonia/respiratory bronchiolitis–interstitial lung disease (DIP/RB–ILD)
- sarcoidosis
- silicosis
- extrinsic allergic alveolitis (EAA)
- pulmonary Langerhans cell histiocytosis (PLCH)
- chronic eosinophilic pneumonia
- alveolar proteinosis
- lymphangitic metastases

- bronchiolitis obliterans with organising pneumonia (BOOP)
- non-specific interstitial pneumonia (NSIP).

Interstitial lung disease (see Fig. 4.11) can be differentiated based on CXR observations. These are listed in Table 4.4.

HRCT indications include equivocally normal CXR, pattern determination and localising the best biopsy site.

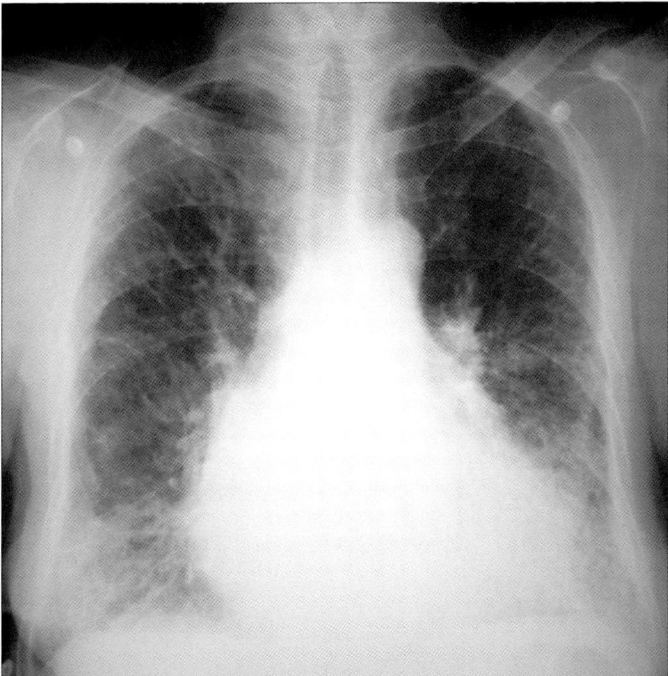

Fig. 4.11 Interstitial fibrosis: PA view

An increase in interstitial shadowing is seen involving all the zones with predominance in the lower zones. At this stage no major volume loss is evident.

It is important to check whether there are signs of previous asbestos exposure, such as pleural calcification. Also check whether there are signs of an erosive arthropathy as rheumatoid arthritis could be a cause. With scleroderma, a dilated oesophagus may be visible.

Interstitial fibrosis is a cause of pulmonary hypertension and right heart failure.

TABLE 4.4 Interstitial lung disease

CXR	Disease
Bibasal involvement	IPF, asbestosis, collagen vascular diseases
Mid and upper lung involvement	Sarcoidosis, silicosis, ankylosing spondylitis, PLCH
Pleural disease	Collagen vascular disease, asbestosis
Hilar lymphadenopathy	Sarcoidosis, malignancy
↓ Lung volumes	Most ILD
Preserved lung volumes	Lympangioleiomyomatosis, PLCH, sarcoidosis
Smokers	DIP, RB-ILD, PLCH

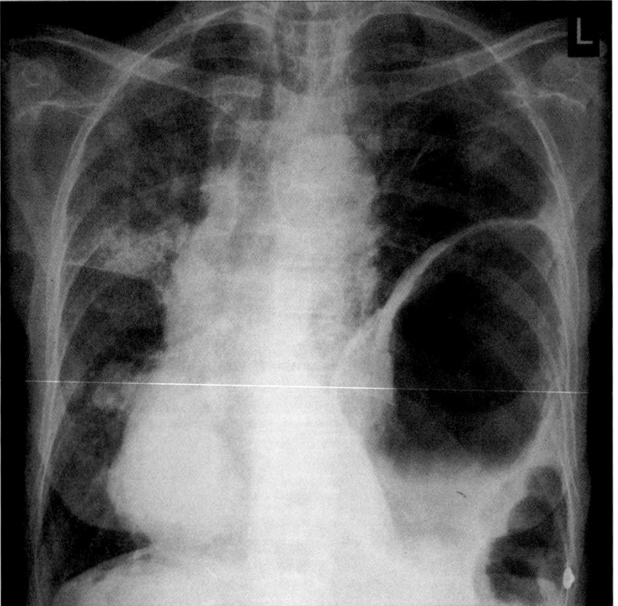

Fig. 4.12 Multiple abnormalities

Two tumours, one small and one large, are seen in the right lower zone and are metastatic deposits. The ground glass opacity seen in the right upper lobe could be due to infection, haemorrhage or tumour obstruction of the right upper lobe bronchus. An unrelated major herniation of the stomach is seen through the left hemidiaphragm.

CHAPTER 5

CARDIOVASCULAR DISORDERS

The chest radiograph is the first and most basic imaging investigation for cardiovascular disorders. There are many other imaging tests available for further cardiac work-up, each with their own indication.

The CXR will help exclude other causes of chest pain (e.g. pneumonia or pneumothorax) if the patient presents to the emergency department. It will not show direct evidence of myocardial ischaemia but may show the effects, e.g. pulmonary oedema.

The heart size and shape need to be assessed first. Remember that a pericardial effusion can mimic cardiomegaly. An enlarged cardiac silhouette and upper lobe blood diversion suggest congestive cardiac failure. Also, it is important to remember that the cardiothoracic ratio is only reliable on posteroanterior (PA) inspiratory films.

The heart shape is abnormal in congenital conditions such as dextrocardia (see Fig. 5.1), tetralogy of Fallot and Ebstein anomaly but it is also important to assess the pulmonary vasculature for evidence of shunts.

Sometimes calcifications are visible in the cardiac shadow. They can occur in the valves, coronary arteries, left ventricular aneurysms (see Fig. 5.2) and in the pericardium. Pericardial calcification often, but not always, correlates with constrictive pericarditis. Atherosclerotic calcifications in the coronary arteries and aorta may be indirect signs of myocardial ischaemia.

Old valve prostheses can sometimes be visible but not the newer prostheses.

All introduced lines and catheters must be checked for their positions. Central lines should pass to the lower superior vena cava (SVC). Pulmonary artery catheters (Swan–Ganz catheters) should not be wedged into small branches. An atrial pacing wire should pass to the lateral wall of the right atrium, whereas the ventricular pacing wire should pass to the apex of the right ventricle. When line and catheter positions are being checked, ensure that there is no iatrogenic pneumothorax (see Chapter 9).

The common cardiovascular disorders are:

- pulmonary oedema
- congestive left heart failure
- pulmonary emboli
- pulmonary artery hypertension
- cor pulmonale
- aortic dissection
- valvular heart disease

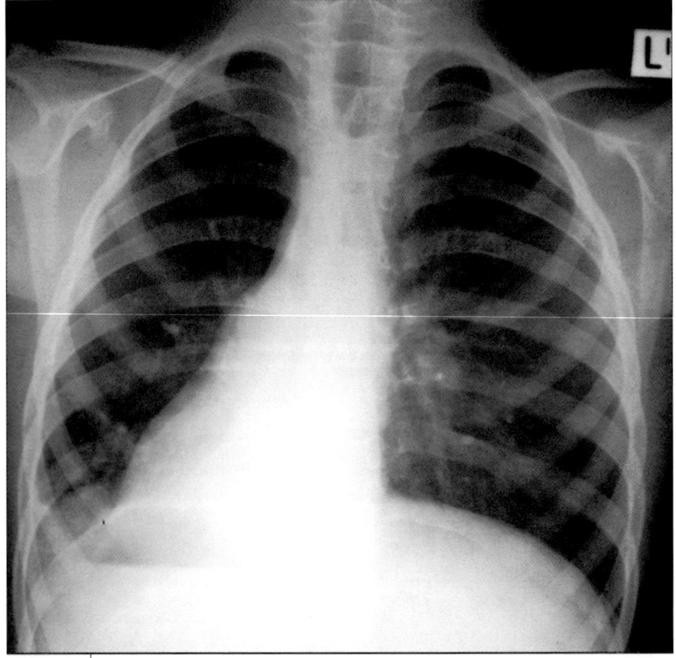

FIG 5.1a

Fig. 5.1 Kartagener syndrome: (a) PA view; (b) bronchogram

The frontal radiograph shows dextrocardia, an increase in markings at the right base due to bronchiectasis and collapse of the right lower lobe (a complication of the bronchiectasis and not part of the syndrome). Please note the gastric air bubble on the right indicating that the dextrocardia is not isolated but part of the situs inversus.

The dilated bronchi are demonstrated on the bronchogram.

Kartagener syndrome is the triad of situs inversus (dextrocardia), bronchiectasis and paranasal sinusitis. About 50% of patients with ciliary dyskinesia have Kartagener syndrome. About 20% of patients with dextrocardia have Kartagener syndrome.

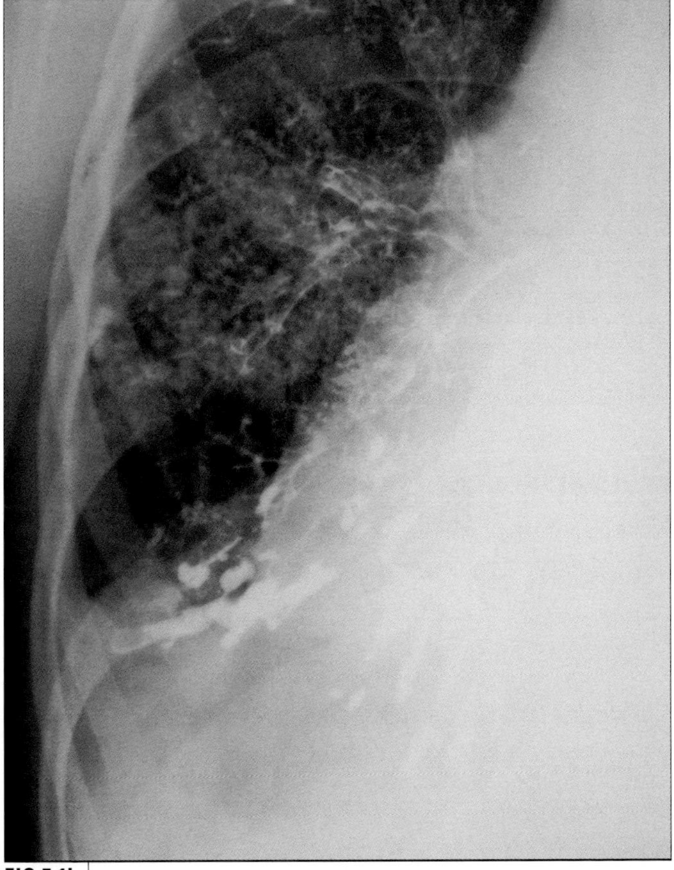

FIG 5.1b

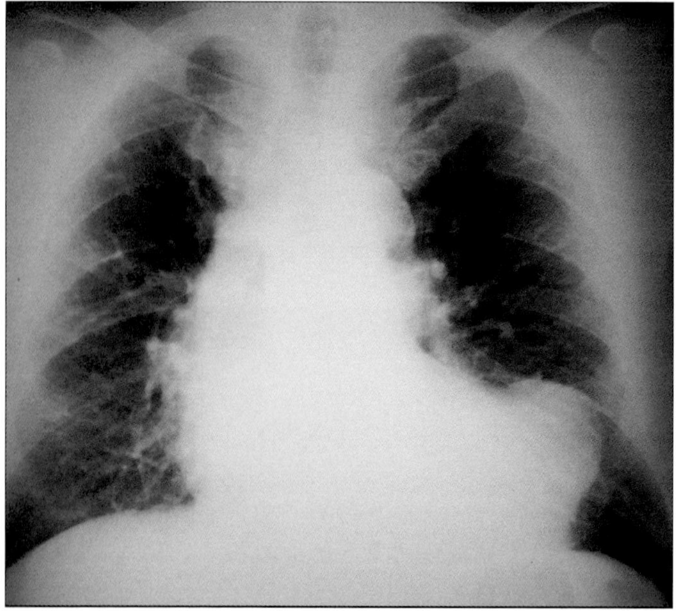

Fig. 5.2 Ventricular aneurysm: PA view

A very prominent bulge is seen on the left heart border due to a ventricular aneurysm. This type of aneurysm usually follows a myocardial infarct and is at risk of rupturing. Differential diagnostic possibilities include localised pericardial defect, cardiac tumour or adjacent pulmonary tumour (see third mogul sign, Appendix 2).

PULMONARY OEDEMA

Pulmonary oedema is the abnormal accumulation of extravascular water in the lung parenchyma.

Normally, there is a net outward filtration of fluid from the lung microvasculature to the perimicrovascular spaces. This small amount of fluid is removed by the pulmonary lymphatic vessels to keep the lungs dry. The lung dryness/wetness status is influenced by:

- capillary blood pressure
- plasma osmotic pressure
- capillary permeability
- alveolar surface tension (surfactant).

Pulmonary oedema is usually due to either elevated pulmonary venous pressure—'**cardiogenic**' oedema—or increased permeability of the alveolar-capillary membrane—'**non-cardiogenic**' oedema. *Hydrostatic pulmonary oedema* is probably a better term than 'cardiogenic' as the main causes are heart disease (increased capillary pressure), over-hydration (aggressive intravenous fluid therapy) or fluid retention (renal failure). In *'non-cardiogenic' pulmonary oedema,* there is some disruption of the capillary endothelium with leakage of fluid into the surrounding lung tissue. However, the oedema fluid is more proteinaceous than in hydrostatic oedema because the capillary injury permits the escape of large molecules as well as fluid.

Although traditionally pulmonary oedema has been classified as being either cardiogenic (hydrostatic) or non-cardiogenic (increased permeability), an even better classification is into four types:

1. hydrostatic
2. permeability oedema without alveolar damage
3. permeability oedema with alveolar damage (ALI, ARDS)
4. mixed hydrostatic and permeability oedema.

Congestive left heart failure

There are a number of causes for congestive left heart failure including myocardial ischaemia, mitral valve disease and aortic valve disease. As the heart fails, it enlarges (cardiomegaly). There is enlargement of the left atrium and left ventricle in mitral regurgitation but only enlargement of the left atrium in mitral stenosis. The left ventricle is enlarged in aortic valve disease. With aortic stenosis, there is aortic valve calcification and post-stenotic dilatation of the aorta. The ascending aorta is also dilated in aortic regurgitation.

There is a typical sequence of changes in the lungs as the left heart fails, from upper zone blood diversion to interstitial pulmonary oedema to alveolar pulmonary oedema.

The normal left atrial pressure or pulmonary venous pressure is less than 12 mmHg. As the heart fails, the pressures rise and produce the typical radiographic changes. The pressure rises in the pulmonary veins can be measured by wedging a pulmonary artery catheter (PAWP).

In the erect position, there is a hydrostatic difference in pressure between the apices and the bases; and in the supine position, between the anterior and posterior aspects. This difference in hydrostatic pressure needs to be added to the pulmonary venous pressure. It also explains why there is more flow to the lower zones and why the first changes occur here. Table 5.1 shows the features of left ventricular failure.

The classic findings in congestive left heart failure are an enlarged heart, widened vascular pedicle and pulmonary venous congestion/oedema. In contrast, the vascular pedicle and heart size are normal

TABLE 5.1	Features of left ventricular failure
• Cardiomegaly (cardiac apex points downwards and outwards)	
• Prominent central pulmonary arteries	
• Signs of upper zone blood diversion and oedema	
• Increase in width of the vascular pedicle	
CXR signs of left atrial enlargement	
• double density sign	
• third (fourth) mogul sign	
• splayed carina 'wishbone' sign	
• posterior bulge of upper cardiac outline (lateral view)	
• displaced barium-filled oesophagus (lateral view)	

in non-cardiogenic pulmonary oedema. Furthermore, if a pulmonary artery catheter wedged pressure is obtained, as for example in intensive care patients, the left atrial pressure is raised in congestive cardiac failure (CCF) (see Table 5.2) and normal in non-cardiogenic pulmonary oedema.

Upper zone blood diversion

In response to the elevated venous pressure (13–17 mmHg), arterial and venous constriction occurs in the lower zones, deviating blood flow to the upper zones (see Fig. 5.3). It is thought that the vasoconstriction is a reaction to early perivascular oedema.

This redistribution of blood flow causes the vessel diameters in the upper zones to be equal to or greater than the comparable lower zone vessels. Also, the upper zone vessels become wider than the

TABLE 5.2	Pulmonary venous wedge pressures in CCF
Radiographic appearance	mmHg
Normal	< 12
Cephalisation of pulmonary vessels	12–17
Kerley lines (interstitial oedema)	> 17
Pleural effusion	> 20
Alveolar oedema	> 25

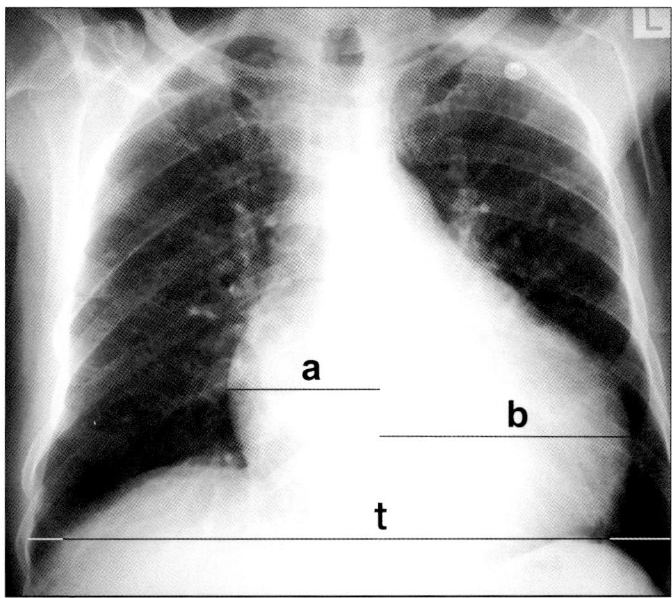

Fig. 5.3 Pulmonary venous congestion: PA view
Compare with Fig. 3.15.

The early sign of left heart failure is the shunting of blood into the upper zone vessels.

The cardiothoracic ratio is the total transverse diameter of the cardiac shadow and the internal diameter of the chest (a + b : t). In this case it is increased above 50%, also indicating that there is left heart failure.

accompanying bronchus (normally the upper zone artery should not exceed its bronchus in diameter). A confirmatory sign is that the vessels projected in the first anterior intercostal space exceed 3 mm in calibre.

Interstitial pulmonary oedema

With a further rise of the pulmonary venous pressure above 17 mmHg, there is leakage of fluid into the interstitium thickening the alveolar walls and interlobular connective tissues. The radiologic signs of interstitial oedema are:

- Kerley lines (oedematous interlobular septa)
- perihilar haze (ground-glass appearance) due to oedema in the extensive interstitial space

- perivascular and peribronchial cuffing
- subpleural fluid accumulation giving the fissures a thickened appearance
- development of a pleural effusion, usually right sided, when the pressure is above 20 mmHg.

The pleural fluid represents transudation of fluid from the visceral pleural surface into the pleural space.

Fig. 5.4 Alveolar pulmonary oedema: (a) PA view; (b) magnified view

The transudate is filling the airspaces and causing the lung to be dense, mainly in a perihilar distribution.

Signs of interstitial pulmonary oedema are also present with transudate thickening the interlobular septa (Kerley B lines). A subpleural or lamellar effusion is also present. The lamellar effusion is a fluid collection in the loose connective tissue beneath the visceral pleura.

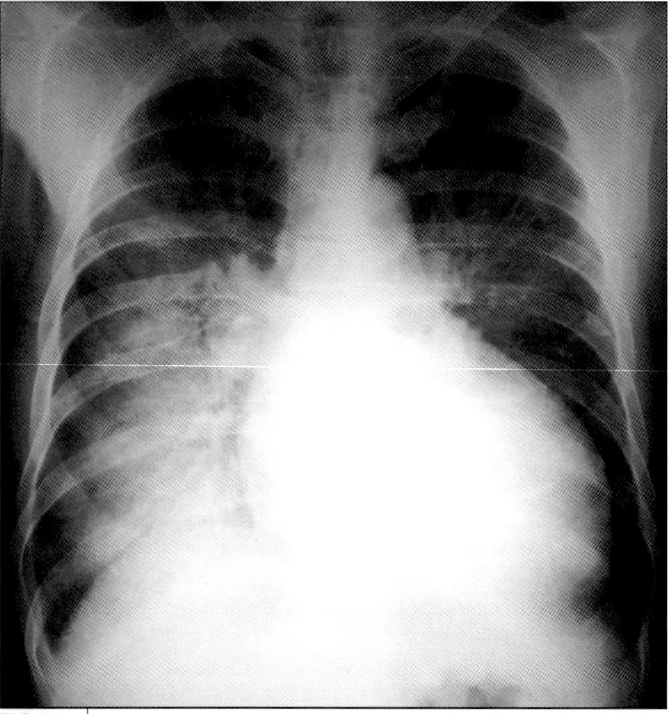

FIG 5.4a

Alveolar pulmonary oedema

When the pulmonary venous pressure rises above 20 mmHg, alveolar oedema fluid spills from the interstitium to the airspaces (see Figs. 5.4, 5.5). Leakage occurs across the previously intact 'tight junctions' of the epithelial basement membrane. The signs of alveolar oedema are:

- confluent non-segmental shadows in a bat's wing/butterfly distribution
- air bronchogram sign (see Appendix 2)
- underlying signs of interstitial oedema.

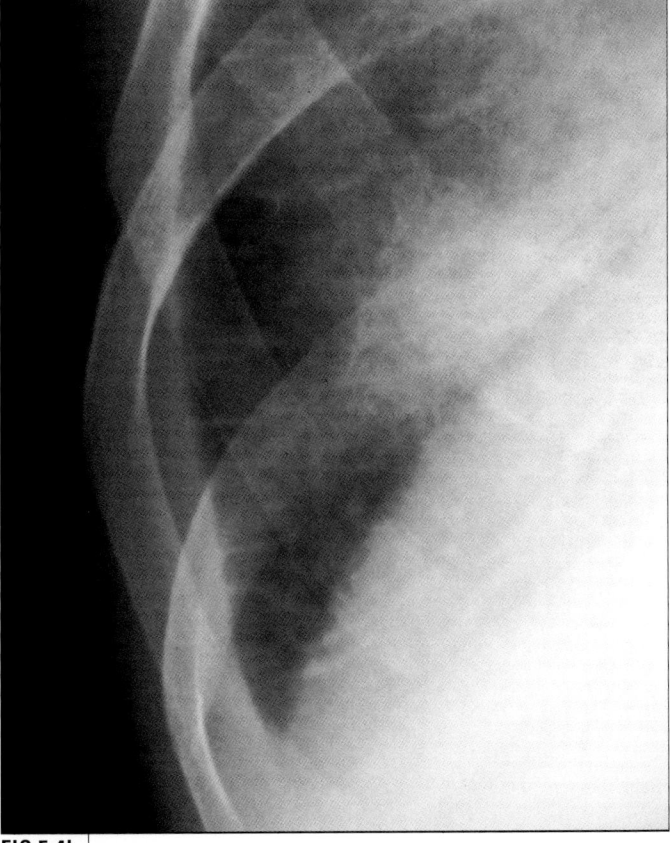

FIG 5.4b

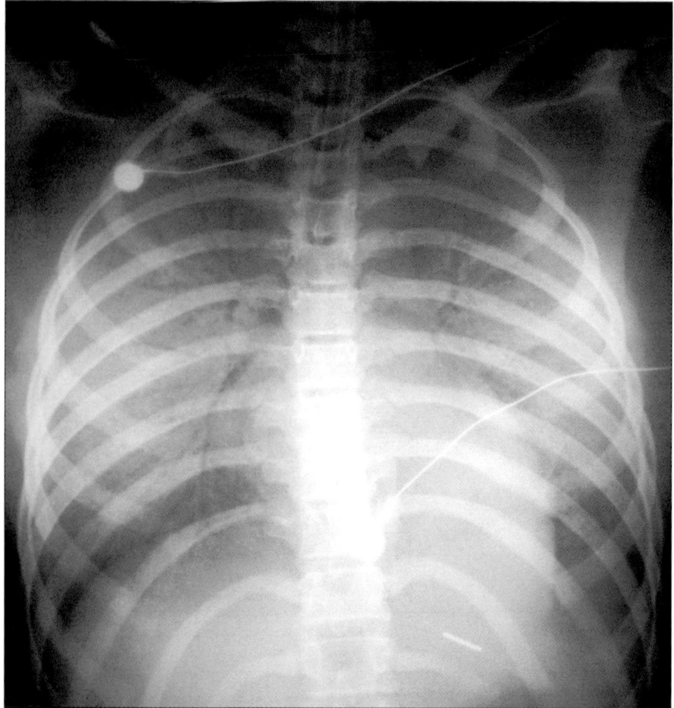

Fig. 5.5 Gross alveolar oedema: AP view

This radiograph shows diffuse and marked airspace filling caused by over-hydration intravenously. Note the normal-sized heart. Air bronchogram signs (see Appendix 2) are well demonstrated.

Airspace filling can be due to transudate (alveolar oedema), exudate (pneumonia), protein (alveolar proteinosis) or cells (alveolar cell carcinoma or lymphoma).

Compartments

The interstitial compartment becomes oedematous first in cardiogenic oedema and therefore may be present without alveolar oedema. However, if alveolar oedema is present, then the interstitial compartment must also be oedematous. Therefore, the signs of alveolar oedema overlay the signs of interstitial oedema.

In increased-permeability oedema, the fluid spills directly into the alveolar spaces and therefore the interstitium may not be oedematous.

Speed of appearance

Flash pulmonary oedema is due to bilateral renal artery stenosis or stenosis in a single functioning kidney. It is characterised by sudden and recurrent episodes of dyspnoea due to the oedema.

Speed of resolution

With treatment, pulmonary oedema can clear rapidly from the lungs. Even so, there can be a 'lag phase' between improving capillary wedge pressure and radiographic resolution. The exception is 'uraemic' pulmonary oedema, which is fibrinous and in which clearing may be very delayed.

Distribution

The distribution of alveolar oedema depends on:

- the patient's posture (e.g. unilateral oedema if the patient is lying on his/her side)
- other lung pathology (e.g. emphysema).

In chronic lung disease there is regional destruction of vasculature with redistribution of blood flow to uninvolved areas which are potential sites for the oedema. Therefore, an 'atypical' distribution is seen.

Central distribution of alveolar oedema occurs because there is more interstitium, a less adequate lymphatic system and less respiratory compression with breathing.

Chronicity

In chronic heart or lung disease, the radiologic changes may occur at higher pressures because of hypertrophy of the lymphatic vessels and adaptations in the microvasculature.

Distinguishing features

Sometimes there are clues to differentiate between cardiogenic and other types of oedema. In cardiogenic oedema, the heart is enlarged and septal lines are common, whereas in increased-permeability oedema the heart size is normal and septal lines are uncommon. In hydrostatic oedema, due to massive intravenous fluid overload, the heart size will not be increased.

Lung volumes

Lung volumes are decreased in pulmonary oedema because of reduced lung compliance.

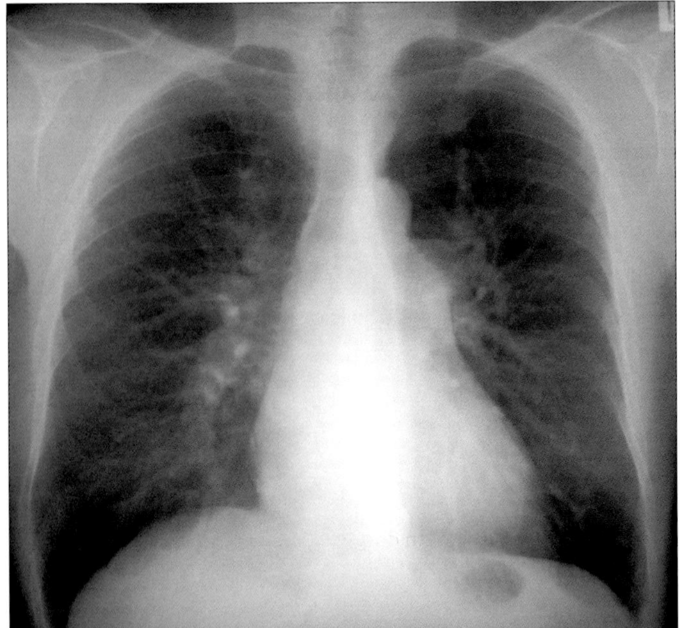

Fig. 5.6 Atrial septal defect (ASD): PA view

In this case of ASD, there is an uncomplicated left-to-right shunt without cardiac enlargement. Enlargement of all the pulmonary vessels, both central and peripheral, in all zones is present, secondary to the increased pulmonary blood flow.

The right heart border (right lateral margin of the right atrium) is prominent. The cardiac apex is becoming elevated, suggesting right ventricular enlargement. The distended pulmonary trunk is causing a bulge below the aortic knuckle. The aortic knuckle is small relative to the pulmonary artery trunk, reflecting the decreased left ventricular output.

Pulmonary arterial over-circulation does not become apparent on chest radiographs until there is a ratio of shunt flow:systemic flow of 2:1. The over-circulation causes pulmonary hypertension when the pressures are greater than 30/15 mmHg (normal pulmonary arterial pressure is 25/10 mmHg). Only with longstanding severe shunts where the pulmonary artery pressure increases above the systemic pressure does reversal of the shunt occur (Eisenmenger syndrome). In Eisenmenger syndrome there is very marked dilatation of the central pulmonary arteries and abrupt pruning of the peripheral arteries as a sign of the increased vascular resistance.

Note that the prominent arteries in this case have sharp margins. This is an important distinguishing feature between a shunt and pulmonary venous hypertension.

Pulmonary embolism

Pulmonary thromboembolism is a common life-threatening condition that is very difficult to diagnose solely on clinical signs and symptoms.

The chest radiograph is abnormal in most cases of pulmonary embolism (PE) but the findings are non-specific, like the clinical signs and symptoms. The non-specific findings that could be present are pleural effusion, atelectasis, parenchymal opacification and elevation of the hemidiaphragm. The classic findings of Hampton hump sign, Westermark sign and Fleischner sign (see Appendix 2) are only rarely seen.

Alternatively, a normal appearing CXR in a patient with severe dyspnoea and hypoxaemia strongly suggests PE if bronchospasm and shunting have been excluded.

Since chest radiography cannot prove or exclude PE conclusively, the radiological work-up of PE requires V/Q isotope scanning, computed tomographic pulmonary angiography (CTPA) and Doppler ultrasound of the legs. The CXR is done routinely with an electrocardiogram (ECG) to identify other diagnoses and to help V/Q scan interpretation. Previously, in difficult cases, pulmonary angiography was required. Nowadays, CT pulmonary angiography is establishing itself as the reference test.

It is important not to exclude the diagnosis of PE based on radiographic evidence of pneumonia or CCF, because these entities may coexist with PE.

Pulmonary artery hypertension

The pressure in the pulmonary artery is dependent on:

- cardiac output (pulmonary artery blood flow)
- cross-sectional area of the pulmonary vasculature
- pulmonary vascular resistance.

Pulmonary arterial hypertension (PAH) is defined as systolic pressure above 25 mmHg (resting) or above 30 mmHg (exercising) or above the mean value of 18 mmHg.

The aetiologies that produce PAH are listed in Appendix 3. The common conditions are chronic pulmonary emboli, CAL, left-to-right shunts and congestive left heart failure.

Pulmonary arterial hypertension needs to be severe before it can be diagnosed on plain films. There is marked enlargement of the pulmonary trunk and hilar pulmonary arteries. The enlargement of the pulmonary trunk causes a prominent convex contour. The enlarged hilar arteries have branches which taper rapidly as they course distally ('pruning'). This discrepancy between the prominent central pulmonary and the narrow peripheral pulmonary arteries is the hallmark sign of pulmonary arterial hypertension. Measurements can be made to confirm PAH. The right interlobar pulmonary artery can be called enlarged (implying PAH) when it is wider than 15 mm in women and 16 mm in men on the PA erect view. The measurement of the left interlobar artery is more difficult to make on the lateral view where 18 mm is the arbitrary division. The pulmonary trunk measurement of above or below 29 mm needs to be made on the CT scan. The enlarged right ventricle is best seen on the lateral view as it impinges into the retrosternal clear space.

The Eisenmenger syndrome or reaction happens when the pulmonary hypertension from a left-to-right shunt becomes so severe that reversal of the shunt occurs. It is associated with polycythaemia and cyanosis.

Cor pulmonale

Cor pulmonale is defined as an alteration in the structure and function of the right ventricle caused by a primary disorder of the respiratory system. Right ventricular disease caused by left heart failure or congenital heart disease is not considered cor pulmonale. Chronic cor pulmonale is commonly caused by COPD and right ventricular hypertrophy predominates.

Acute cor pulmonale is most commonly due to massive pulmonary embolism and produces right ventricular dilatation.

On chest radiography, there will be signs of the underlying lung disease, signs of pulmonary hypertension, and dilated right heart chambers. The transverse diameter of the heart may increase and on the lateral view there is filling of the retrosternal air space.

AORTIC DISSECTION

Aortic dissection is a medical and surgical emergency with many patients presenting with acute chest pain. The chest X-ray is useful if it suggests findings consistent with aortic dissection or is suggestive of other causes. However, in 25% of patients the CXR may be normal, e.g. the widened ascending aorta is hidden within the mediastinal shadow. If there is a high clinical suspicion of dissection, a CT aortogram or transoesophageal echocardiogram (TOE) is urgently indicated.

The CXR signs of aortic dissection are:

- widened superior mediastinum
- wide ascending, arch or descending aorta

- widened or deformed aortic knob
- displaced intimal calcification
- enlarged cardiac shadow (AI or haemopericardium)
- pleural effusion, usually on left
- apical cap (extrapleural haematoma).

Aortic dissections have been subdivided by the Stanford and DeBakey classifications to facilitate surgical decision making. Stanford type A aortic dissections involves the ascending aorta and may (DeBakey type I) or may not (DeBakey type II) involve the arch.

VALVULAR HEART DISEASE

The general signs of valvular heart disease such as cardiomegaly, particular chamber enlargement, apex displacement, and pulmonary signs of left heart failure, are important observations on the CXR. However, with TOE and other tests, the subtle and variable signs of particular valvular disease are not important.

Enlargement of the left atrium indicates mitral stenosis (MS) or mitral incompetence (MI). The left ventricle will also be enlarged on MI. Radiographic signs of mitral valve disease include:

- double contour sign
- splaying of the carina
- mitralisation of the left heart border due to dilatation of the left atrial appendage (third mogul sign)
- posterior displacement of the upper posterior margin of the heart. In previous years this was shown on the lateral CXR by a barium-filled oesophagus.
- pulmonary signs of left heart failure, i.e. blood redistribution and pulmonary oedema
- pulmonary haemosiderosis.

CHAPTER 6

PLEURAL ABNORMALITIES

On a normal chest radiograph, the pleural space is an invisible compartment. With disease, pleural abnormalities become visible. Recognition and understanding of these pleural abnormalities is needed for correct CXR interpretation.

The common pleural abnormalities are:

- pneumothorax
- pleural effusion
- empyema
- pseudotumour
- mesothelioma
- rounded atelectasis
- pleural plaques/diffuse pleural thickening
- fibrothorax
- apical capping.

PNEUMOTHORAX

Pneumothorax is air in the pleural space. It may occur spontaneously or result from a traumatic cause. If small it may have only subtle signs and be difficult to diagnose. Subtle signs of a pneumothorax in a supine patient are the anterior sulcus sign, deep sulcus sign and 'double diaphragm' sign (see Appendix 2). A tension pneumothorax (see Figure 6.1) is a medical emergency.

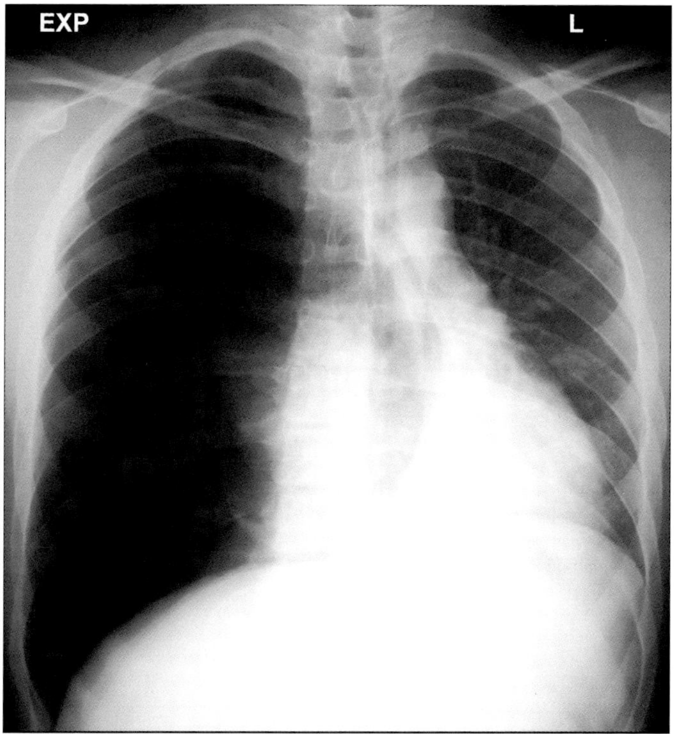

Fig. 6.1 Tension pneumothorax: PA view

Tension pneumothorax is a medical emergency. Therefore, clinical or radiological recognition is very important. Clinically, these patients are hypoxic with haemodynamic collapse.

The classic features demonstrated in this case are the shift of the trachea and mediastinum to the left, depression of the right hemidiaphragm and compression of the right lung. The markedly increased translucent right pleural space projects beyond the midline into the left hemithorax.

The air leak is through a tear, which behaves like a valve. The air leaks out on inspiration due to negative pleural pressure and is then under tension in the neutral and expiratory phases.

Paradoxically, the density of the collapsing lung changes very little because the blood flow diminishes in parallel.

If the underlying lung is stiff or consolidated, there can be significant tension, even if little lung collapse is present.

Drainage of a tension pneumothorax may result in an uncommon complication of re-expansion pulmonary oedema.

Primary spontaneous pneumothorax

These pneumothoraces occur in apparently healthy individuals (primary) and without a traumatic cause (spontaneous). The male/female ratio is 6:1 and typically occurs between 20 and 40 years of age. It is usually due to rupture of an apical pleural bleb.

Secondary spontaneous pneumothorax

These pneumothoraces develop in patients with predisposing lung or pleural disease without a precipitating traumatic event. COPD is the most common cause. Any patient with underlying pulmonary fibrosis is at risk. Other causes include cavitating neoplasms, Marfan syndrome or pleural endometriosis (catamenial).

Traumatic pneumothorax

Traumatic pneumothorax can develop with either penetrating or closed chest trauma. Closed chest trauma or blunt chest trauma can produce a pneumothorax by laceration of airways, fractured ribs causing laceration of the lungs, or by alveolar disruption due to increased intra-thoracic pressure.

Iatrogenic pneumothorax

Pneumothorax is a not infrequent complication of medical procedures such as central venous catheter insertion and lung biopsy.

In ventilated patients, it is important that even small pneumothoraces are recognised as they can quickly progress to life-threatening tension pneumothoraces.

PLEURAL EFFUSIONS

A variety of diseases can cause fluid to enter and accumulate in the pleural space. This fluid can be a transudate, exudate, pus, blood or chyle. Radiographically, the contents cannot be distinguished. Other terminology may be used if the contents are known, e.g. haemothorax, chylothorax, empyema (pyothorax) and hydropneumothorax.

Transudates and exudates can be separated biochemically by their protein content. Transudative effusions have a low protein content, < 50% of the serum protein, usually < 3 g/litre. Transudates form when there is a shift in Starling forces across the pleural capillaries with either an increase in hydrostatic pressure or a decrease in colloid osmotic pressure. Transudates tend to be bilateral and are not associated with pleural disease. Exudative effusions form when there is increased permeability of the pleural capillaries because of inflammatory or malignant processes.

In the absence of trauma and surgery, a haemorrhagic pleural effusion raises the suspicion of a malignant process.

When the patient is supine, any free pleural fluid layers out posteriorly. The best sign on the supine AP radiograph is the reduced translucency of the lung.

Pleural effusion usually creates a characteristic homogeneous opacity with a meniscal margin on the erect chest radiograph (see meniscal sign, Appendix 2). Being heavier than the air-filled lung, the fluid collects between the hemidiaphragm and the lung base with loss of visualisation of the hemidiaphragm (see silhouette sign, Appendix 2). No lung or air bronchograms should be seen. The lung retracts from the chest wall parietal pleura but less so from the mediastinal surface. This lung is passively collapsed.

A subpulmonary effusion is more common on the right than the left but can be bilateral. Subpulmonic fluid lifts the lung base away from the hemidiaphragm and can mimic a raised hemidiaphragm. On a PA erect projection, the peak of the pseudo diaphragmatic configuration is lateral to that of the normal hemidiaphragm. If the subpulmonary effusion is on the left, there is an increase in the distance between the gastric fundus and lung base of more than 2 cm.

Decubitus films will show if the fluid is free-flowing or loculated. Subpulmonary effusions are mobile and will move to the gravity dependent position on decubitus films.

If there are interpleural fibrinous adhesions, the fluid can loculate in the fissures or elsewhere in the pleural space. Sometimes this loculated pleural fluid (encysted) can mimic a mass—called a 'pseudotumour' or 'phantom' tumour.

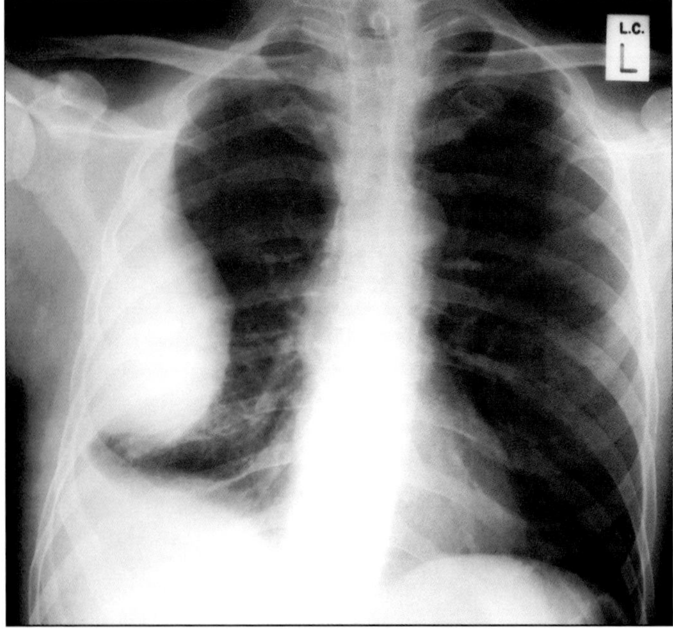

Fig. 6.2 Loculated pleural effusion: PA view

There is a large, right pleural-based opacity. Its shape indicates that it is externally loculated and by inference there are also internal loculations formed. Its upper edge is seen to taper into the pleural margin. Associated elevation of the right hemidiaphragm (subpulmonanry effusion) and blunting of the right costophrenic angle are also seen.

No rib erosion or evidence of osteomyelitis is present to suggest spread of either possible tumour or infection.

In the appropriate clinical setting with fever, this pleural loculation could be an empyema.

Confirmation that this is loculated pleural fluid could be established by ultrasound or CT scanning. (See D sign, Appendix 2.)

EMPYEMA

Exudative effusions commonly loculate, and more so with haemothorax. An empyema is an infected loculated exudative collection in the pleural space which, if untreated, progresses to a frankly purulent collection with pleural thickening.

Pleural fluid begins to accumulate first in the posterior costophrenic angle which is the most gravity dependent portion of the pleural space in the upright patient. About 150 mL of pleural fluid will be the first sign of blunting of the posterior costophrenic angle.

More pleural fluid, about 200 mL will be needed before blunting of the lateral costophrenic angles will be visualised on the frontal film.

In large pleural effusions, inversion of the hemidiaphragm may occur. It is more likely on the left than the right where there is liver support. Even following successful thoracocentesis, the height of the meniscus may be unchanged because the diaphragmatic inversion has reversed.

Special effusions

- Large unilateral pleural effusions should raise the possibilities of infection, tumour, haemorrhage or chyle.
- If an effusion becomes very large, it can cause a 'white-out' of the hemithorax. Typically, there is mediastinal shift to the contralateral side but this may not happen because of the accompanying compression atelectasis. If a tension hydrothorax develops, there is a marked mediastinal displacement and haemodynamic compromise.
- As well as the usual causes, a left-only pleural effusion can be typical of pancreatitis (elevated pleural fluid amylase) and oesophageal rupture (fluid contains salivary amylase) and tears of the upper part of the thoracic duct. Left-only pleural effusion is also seen in aortic dissection.
- Lamellar effusion, as is seen in CCF, is not in the pleural space but is accumulated fluid in the subvisceral connective tissue. This space is in continuity with the interlobular septa and there often are Kerley B lines (see Figure 5.4).
- 'Wet pleura' is thickening of the interlobar fissures and is commonly seen in CCF. This thickening is due to early or residual traces of fluid in the pleural spaces and oedema in the subpleural connective tissue.
- Sympathetic effusion is an exudative pleural effusion caused by an inflammatory response to a disease in a nearby structure (subdiaphragmatic abscess, pneumonia, pericarditis, pancreatitis). This pleural fluid may or may not be infected.
- Parapneumonic effusion arises in nearly half of bacterial pneumonias. Three types may occur: exudative and non-infected (uncomplicated), exudative and infected (complicated) and empyema.
- Pleural effusions due to liver cirrhosis occur because of ascitic fluid leak through the diaphragm and also decreased serum albumin levels.

- Chylous pleural effusions (chylothorax) are usually due to thoracic duct transection by trauma or surgery, or malignant obstruction of the thoracic duct, often lymphoma. They are turbid or milky in appearance and contain chylomicrons.
- Pseudochylous effusions or chyliform effusions are rich in cholesterol and contain no chylomicrons. Typically they have a fat-fluid level. They are often chronic post-inflammatory effusions.
- Unusual effusions are due to bile (bilothorax), urine, ascitic fluid, peritoneal dialysate or CSF (ventriculopleural shunt).
- In Meigs syndrome, there is a pleural effusion associated with a benign ovarian tumour and ascites.
- Catamenial haemothorax is recurrent haemothorax occurring with the menses and due to pleurodiaphragmatic endometriosis.
- Benign pleural effusions can occur as a manifestation of asbestos-related pleural disease. However, effusions often accompany mesothelioma,
- Empyema necessitans (necessitatis) is a rare complication of empyema where there is extension of the infection through the chest wall and percutaneous drainage.

PSEUDOTUMOUR

A pseudotumour produces a curious, rather than spurious, shadow on the frontal film resembling a pulmonary mass but on the lateral film has a lenticular or cigar shape. It is due to loculated (encysted) fluid in a pleural fissure (see Fig. 6.3). They are usually seen with congestive cardiac failure and resolve with treatment. They are also called vanishing or phantom tumours (see lemon sign, Appendix 2).

Pleural tumours

Metastatic disease is the most common pleural tumour. Mesothelioma is the primary malignant tumour of the pleura with three histological types: epithelial, mesenchymal and mixed. Pleura sarcomas are rare. Benign tumours are the fibrous tumour of the pleura and pleural lipoma.

Fig. 6.3 Pseudotumour (a) PA view; (b) lateral view

The right mid-zone opacity is due to loculated pleural fluid in the upper oblique fissure. Such a pseudotumour is more likely to occur in patients with a history of cardiac failure. Small effusions are blunting the posterior costophrenic angles.

There are two pacemaker leads; one passing to the right atrial appendage and the other passing to the apex of the right ventricle.

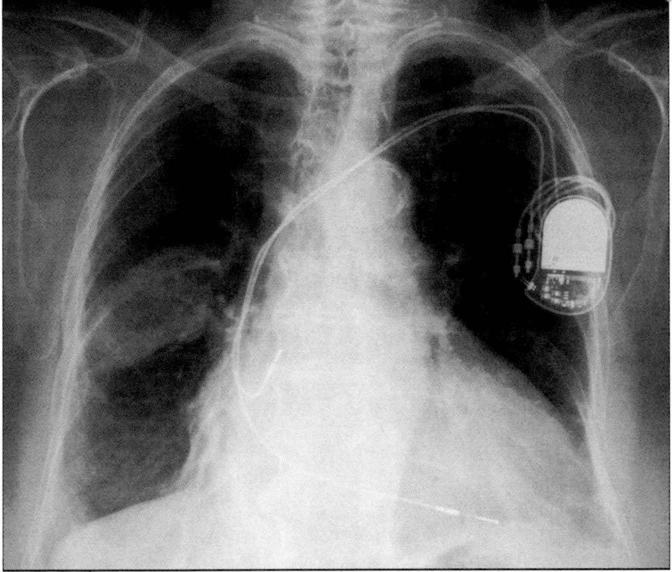

FIG 6.3a

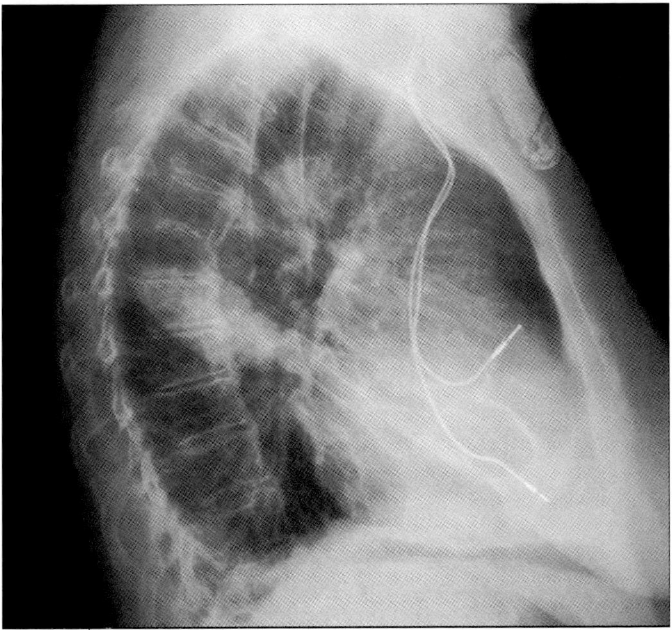

FIG 6.3b

Fibrous tumour of the pleura

Pathologists prefer the description of solitary (or localised) fibrous tumour of the pleura rather than pleural fibroma. Benign mesothelioma is a term that should *not* be used as the tumour actually arises from the submesothelial connective tissue and also the tumour is not always benign.

About 50% are pedunculated and may be difficult to biopsy percutaneously because of their mobility. Because of the possibility of malignancy, excision and long-term surveillance is necessary. They are an interesting pathology because of possible associated hypertrophic pulmonary osteoarthropathy (HPOA) and the Doege-Potter syndrome.

MESOTHELIOMA

Mesothelioma is a primary pleural neoplasm that arises from the mesothelial cells.

About 80% of cases occur where there is an occupational history of exposure to asbestos, e.g. construction, shipyard and insulation industries. In Australia, the UK and Europe the incidence will not peak until 2020, due to the continuing use of asbestos until the 1980s and the latency period of at least 20 years. The USA has probably passed its peak incidence.

The tumour grows along the pleural spaces, including the fissures, as nodular thickening and may even encase the lung circumferentially. It can then invade the mediastinum and beyond the diaphragm.

Metastatic adenocarcinoma causing diffuse pleural thickening can mimic the appearance of mesothelioma. The pathologist needs to perform special stains and election microscopy to differentiate adenocarcinoma from the epithelial type of mesothelioma. The radiologist must look for clues of asbestos exposure, such as calcified pleural plaques.

ROUNDED ATELECTASIS

Rounded atelectasis is also known as round atelectasis, atelectatic pseudotumour, helical atelectasis, Blesovsky syndrome and folded lung.

Rounded atelectasis is a mass-like opacity, usually between 2–7 cm in diameter that appears round on the CXR. However, on CT it has more of a comet tail appearance (see comet tail sign, Appendix 2) due to the convergence of vessels into the atelectatic mass. There is thickening and retraction of the visceral pleura such that the subpleural atelectatic lung develops a rounded configuration.

Although there are several causes, the majority are due to asbestos exposure. The diagnostic clue is asbestos-induced pleural plaques associated with the mass-like opacity. However, biopsy may be necessary in atypical appearances because of the increased risk of bronchogenic carcinoma in asbestos-exposed workers.

The commonest position for this opacity is on the posterior aspect of the lower lobes.

PLEURAL PLAQUES

Pleural plaques are the commonest manifestation and best indicator of asbestos exposure. The plaques more commonly occur on the parietal pleura and are composed of collagen. These plaques can calcify and may produce a holly-leaf appearance when viewed enface (see Fig. 6.4). If they are situated over the pericardial surface they can produce the 'shaggy heart' sign (see Appendix 2).

When pleural plaques are identified they indicate asbestos exposure but not asbestosis, which is the interstitial fibrosis.

Fig. 6.4 Calcified pleural plaques

Multiple bizarrely shaped calcifications are seen bilaterally consistent with asbestos-induced calcified pleural plaques, sometimes resembling a holly leaf in shape. There is no overt asbestosis (interstitial fibrosis).

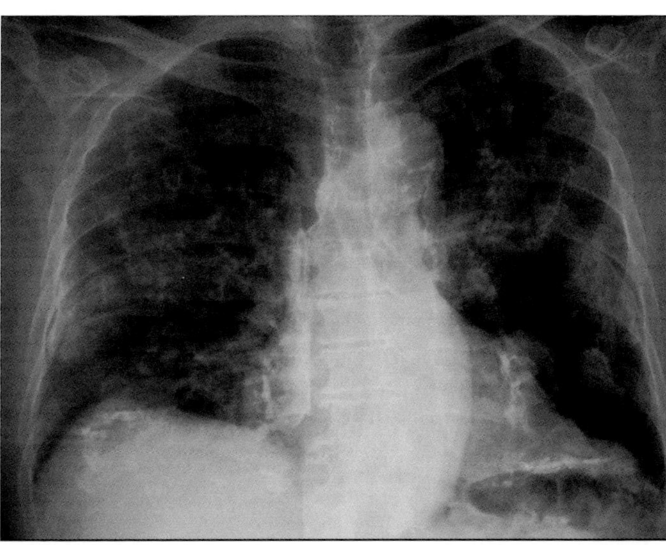

Diffuse pleural thickening

Diffuse pleural thickening is extensive plaque formation which may differ from the diffuse thickening seen following benign asbestos-related pleural effusion. The clinical significance of diffuse pleural thickening is that it may encase enough of the lung to cause 'restrictive' lung function, mimicking asbestosis.

FIBROTHORAX

Fibrothorax is literally fibrosis of the pleural space. An extensive rind of pleural thickening (pleural peel) occurs following a chronic empyema. It is on the outer surfaces but not the mediastinal surface. The lung volume is reduced ('trapped lung') and the hemithorax narrowed. The parietal and visceral pleura become thickened and usually calcify (see Fig. 4.4 on page 77). Thickened fibrous material and/or fluid is seen in the pleural space. The overlying extrapleural fat becomes thickened.

APICAL PLEURAL THICKENING

An 'apical cap' is often due to subpleural scarring and this is more commonly seen in elderly patients. Although often thought to be due to granulomatous scarring from tuberculosis, it usually is non-granulomatous post-inflammatory scarring (see differential diagnosis of apical pleural thickening in Appendix 3). In acute and traumatic settings, for example, in aortic dissection, the capping could be extrapleural dissection of mediastinal blood.

TABLE 6.1 Pulmonary and pleural asbestos diseases
• pleural plaques
• benign asbestos-related pleural effusion
• diffuse pleural thickening
• rounded area of atelectasis
• asbestosis
• mesothelioma
• lung carcinoma

CHAPTER 7

MEDIASTINAL MALADIES

MEDIASTINAL MASSES

A mediastinal mass visibly declares itself on the chest radiograph as an opacity bulging from a normal mediastinal outline and displacing the lung. More subtle findings include displacement or narrowing of the trachea, the carina, or a contrast-filled oesophagus.

For radiological description and as an aid to the differential diagnoses, the mass needs to be identified as occupying a particular mediastinal compartment (see Figure 7.1) but this can become complicated by the different versions of the divisions.

Anterior mediastinal mass

The differential diagnosis of an anterior mediastinal mass is best remembered by the 5 Ts (see Appendix 3), i.e. thyroid, thymus, teratoma, terrible lymphoma and tortuous vessel. A bronchogenic carcinoma lying against the mediastinal margin could simulate a mediastinal mass.

Most thyroid masses are due to colloid nodular goitres but occasionally can be due to carcinoma or lymphoma. Large thyroid masses extend downwards into the mediastinum and are not always typically 'retrosternal'.

There are several thymic abnormalities: they may present as an anterior mediastinal mass, including thymoma, thymic hyperplasia, thymic carcinoid, thymic carcinoma, thymic cyst, thymic lymphoma and thymolipoma.

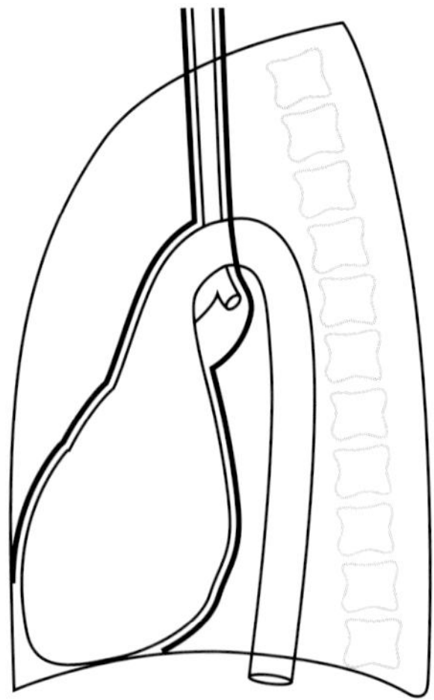

Fig. 7.1 Mediastinal compartments (anterior, middle and posterior)
This version has the pericardium and its contents in the middle mediastinum but, unlike the traditional anatomical version, dispenses with the superior mediastinum.

Superiorly the more anterior vascular structures are included in the anterior mediastinum.

Teratoma in the '5T' differential diagnosis (see Appendix 3), for simplicity, represents primary germ cell tumours. These also include dermoid cyst, seminoma, choriocarcinoma, embryonal cell carcinoma and yolk sac tumours. They arise from rests of primitive germ cells that were left in the mediastinum during their fetal migration from the yolk sac to the urogenital ridge. Teratomas represent at least 50% of all mediastinal germ cell tumours. There is usually mature or immature tissue derived from the three germinal layers (ectoderm, endoderm and mesoderm).

CT scanning is the best modality for identifying calcification and fat densities within the anterior mediastinal mass that may indicate that it is a germ cell neoplasm.

Middle mediastinal mass

If a middle mediastinal mass is identified, it is usually due to lymphadenopathy (neoplastic, inflammatory or infectious). However,

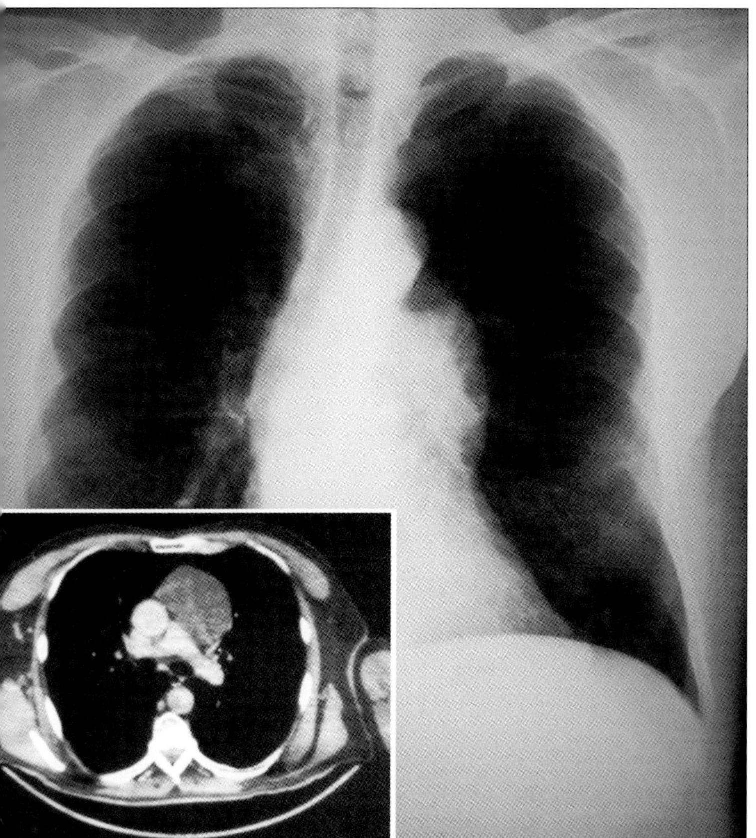

Fig. 7.2 Anterior mediastinal mass (plus inset)
There is an opacity projected over the left hilum. The left hilum is still visualised (hilar overlay sign) indicating that the mass is either anterior or posterior to the hilum. In this case, it is due to a thymic cyst (anterior mediastinal mass).

other considerations are a bronchogenic cyst, pericardial cyst or a vascular abnormality.

Signs of calcification within the mass can be confirmed on CT scanning and may narrow the differential diagnoses.

Secondary effects of mediastinal lymphadenopathy are pulmonary lymphangitis carcinomatosis and SVC obstruction.

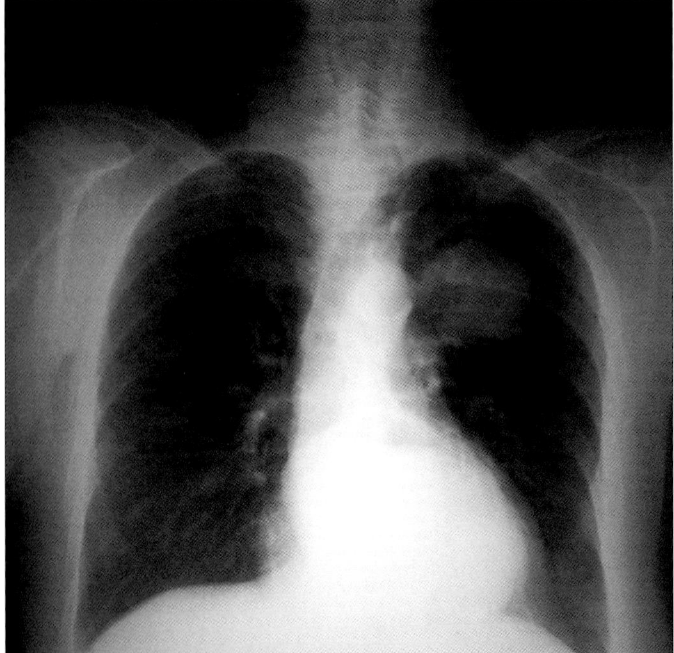

Fig. 7.3 Goitre, lung tumour and hiatus hernia
Three abnormalities are present: the trachea is deviated by a goitre; a 5 cm mass is seen in the left upper zone and a large hiatus hernia is seen behind the heart.

Posterior mediastinal mass

The normal structures in the posterior mediastinum are the descending aorta, oesophagus and thoracic spine, which can all produce abnormal masses. Descending aortic aneurysm, oesophageal mass, oesophageal duplication cyst and paravertebral masses need to be considered. Remember that many posterior mediastinal masses are neurogenic in origin.

Paravertebral masses

The thoracic spine is the posterior border of the mediastinum, but all the paravertebral soft tissues are often included in posterior mediastinum compartment in the different classifications.

Lateral paravertebral masses will cause displacement of the paraspinal stripe.

Neurogenic tumours, extramedullary haemopoesis, paravertebral haematomas and spondylodiscitis inflammatory mass are in the differential diagnoses.

Acute mediastinitis

The plain radiograph may have little to add in the diagnosis of acute mediastinitis where a high clinical suspicion is needed. The most common cause is iatrogenic oesophageal perforation at endoscopy. Pneumomediastinum may be a radiological clue. More rarely, Boerhaave syndrome is spontaneous oesophageal perforation.

Acute mediastinitis can occur post-operatively after median sternotomy for cardiothoracic surgery. Mediastinal leakage after perforation by central venous catheters is another cause.

Fibrosing mediastinitis

Fibrosing mediastinitis is usually caused by a chronic granulomatous infection, mostly commonly histoplasmosis and tuberculosis. It could be that the fibro-inflammatory response is immunological rather than direct infection. The scarring can cause compression of the SVC, central airways, central pulmonary vessels or oesophagus.

The chest radiograph can show non-specific widening of the mediastinum. Calcified mediastinal lymph nodes may be observed.

The proximal pulmonary veins may be compressed and produce a clinical syndrome similar to mitral stenosis.

Pneumomediastinum

As the name indicates, pneumomediastinum is the condition where gas lies in the connective tissue planes of the mediastinum (see Fig. 7.4). The most common cause is dissection of air from alveolar rupture along the bronchovascular bundles to the mediastinum. Less frequent causes are oesophageal and the tracheobronchial perforation and extension of free air from the neck or abdomen. Gas forming infection is a rare cause (see causes of pneumomediastinum, Appendix 3).

The CXR shows lucent streaks and gas bubbles along the mediastinal contours and also in the superior mediastinum extending towards the neck. The continuous diaphragm sign and the V sign of Naclerio may be other clues that a pneumomediastinum is present. The 'angel wing' sign indicates gas around the thymus in a neonate. On the lateral view, the translucencies are most easily seen in the retrosternal region. If air lies around the right pulmonary artery, it is known as 'ring around the artery' sign.

Pneumopericardium can be distinguished from pneumomediastinum by the confinement of the gas to the pericardial sac. On decubitus views, the pneumomediastinal gas will be unchanged but gas in the pneumopericardium will rise to the non-dependent side of the heart.

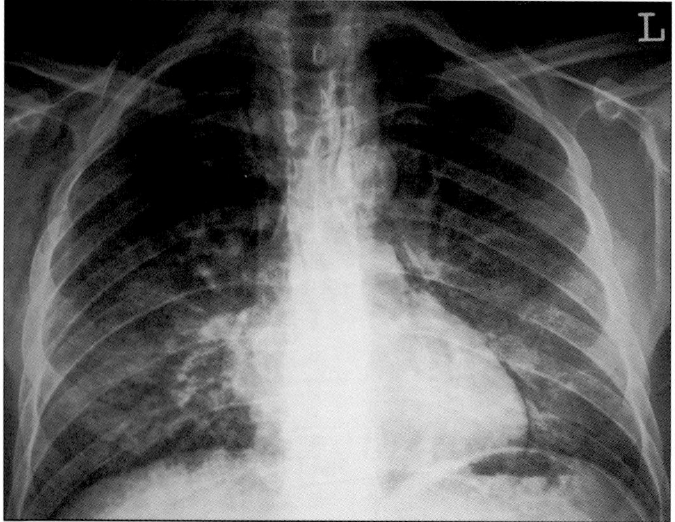

Fig. 7.4 Pneumomediastinum

Streaky lucencies are seen around the left cardiac margin and within the superior mediastinum. Subcutaneous gas is seen over the right chest wall.

The mild diffuse change in the lungs is due to pneumocystis infection. As with any pneumonia, the coughing has produced alveolar rupture with air dissection into the mediastinum (Macklin effect). Similarly, raised alveolar pressure which can induce alveolar rupture can occur with vomiting and the Valsalva manoeuvre.

CHAPTER 8

CHEST TRAUMA

Chest trauma is second only to head trauma as a cause of trauma-related death. Blunt trauma and penetrating trauma have different mechanisms of injury and manifestations.

Blunt chest trauma is frequently due to motor vehicle accidents and falls from heights. Rapid deceleration and direct external blows can result in significant injuries to the chest wall, lung and mediastinum.

With penetrating injury, the entry site of injury is usually known, e.g. knife wound or gunshot wound, although the direction of the trajectory may be difficult to predict. With an epigastric penetration, it is difficult to tell clinically whether the injury is above or below the diaphragm, or both. The major risk is to the mediastinal vascular structures or lung laceration causing a tension pneumothorax.

The chest X-ray is the first imaging study in chest trauma. The easily performed mobile CXR can expedite treatments in the emergency department before a CT scan is performed. Remember that aortic injury, cardiac tamponade and tension pneumothorax are the most immediate life-threatening conditions. Many of the traumatic injuries are better seen on the CT scan than the CXR alone.

CHEST WALL INJURY

Bony injuries include rib fractures, sternal fractures, spinal fractures, clavicular fractures and sternoclavicular joint dislocations.

Beware of fractures of the costal cartilages or disrupted costochondral junctions, which will not be recognised on radiographs but still may contribute to a flail chest.

Surgical emphysema is gas in the subcutaneous tissue of the chest wall. It could be due to a penetrating lung injury or an extension of a pneumomediastinum or pneumothorax.

Rib fracture

Isolated rib fracture with minimal displacement is unlikely to change clinical management. Therefore, some have proposed that a frontal CXR is sufficient to rule out significant rib fractures without the need to perform oblique views. Undisplaced fractures may be seen on these oblique views as a step in the cortical edge.

More serious is the 'flail chest' which has varying definitions (see Glossary). It can be due to fractures of several adjacent ribs or two fractures in each of at least three adjacent ribs. There is also, invariably, underlying pleural and lung injury. The flail chest will cause respiratory compromise because of the combination of paradoxical movement during respiration and the underlying lung injury.

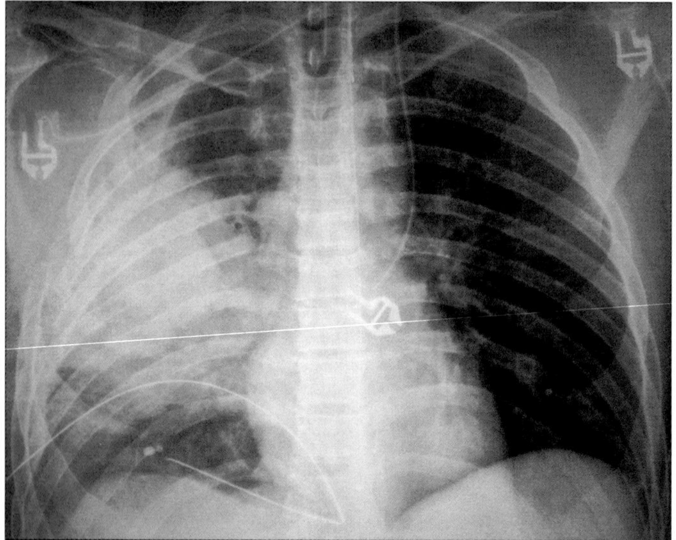

Fig. 8.1 Chest trauma

Multiple fractured right ribs are seen with associated haemothorax and lung contusion. Further imaging of the right clavicle and scapula will be necessary to assess their suspected injuries.

The right basal chest drain is kinked at the inferomedial pleural corner.

The endotracheal tube is too high.

'Stove-in' chest is the variant of flail chest where there is inward deformity of the flail segment and compression of the thoracic contents. It is associated with a high mortality unless corrected.

The first three ribs are partially protected by the shoulders and scapulae. Therefore fractures here usually indicate severe trauma. The subclavian vessels may be injured following fractures to the clavicle or first rib. Brachial plexus injury also needs to be considered following a first rib injury.

Fractures to the lower ribs may be associated with injuries to the liver, kidneys and spleen.

In children, the ribs are more supple and less likely to fracture but there may be underlying lung contusion.

SPINAL FRACTURE

Most vertebral injuries are produced by hyperflexion and/or axial loading occurring mostly at the T9–T11 levels. Look for vertebral malalignment, malalignment of the posterior elements and paraspinal line thickening/haematoma.

Compression fractures can be identified on the lateral CXR as well as on dedicated thoracic spine X-rays.

The more serious vertebral fracture-dislocation has a high chance of being associated with a spinal cord injury.

Pneumorachis (air in the spinal canal) is a very rare sign following trauma.

STERNAL FRACTURE

Sternal fractures can result from steering wheel injury, seat-belt injury and cardiopulmonary resuscitation.

A sternal fracture and sternoclavicular joint dislocation may be missed on the frontal film. The lateral CXR will better show the sternum and even oblique views may be helpful. A lateral 'shoot-through' view may be required if the patient cannot be moved from the supine position.

PULMONARY PARENCHYMAL INJURY

These are lung contusion, laceration or frank haematoma.

Lung contusion appears as consolidation which resolves over a few days.

Lung laceration is invariably associated with a pneumothorax. A late manifestation of lung laceration may be a pneumatocoele (an ovoid translucency).

PLEURAL ABNORMALITY

Pleural abnormalities, i.e. pneumothorax and pleural effusion (haemothorax) are a common association with injuries to the chest wall, lung and mediastinum.

Remember that trauma patients are radiographed in the supine position and that pneumothorax and haemothorax will look different from that seen on an erect position radiograph. An erect CXR may not be possible until major spinal injuries have been excluded. The free air in a supine pneumothorax will accumulate in the non-dependent portion of the pleural space, i.e. anteriorly over the lower chest (see the deep sulcus sign, anterior sulcus sign and the 'double diaphragm' sign, Appendix 2). Besides the prominent lateral costophrenic angle and basal lucency, there may be an unusually sharp delineation of the mediastinal contour. Even a small pneumothorax is important to identify because it may increase to a tension pneumothorax on positive pressure ventilation.

A tension pneumothorax is a medical emergency and requires immediate recognition and treatment.

The majority of pleural collections following trauma are due to haemorrhage. A rapidly expanding pleural effusion is most likely arterial in origin, e.g. laceration of intercostal, internal mammary or mediastinal arteries.

DIAPHRAGMATIC RUPTURE

Diaphragmatic rupture can occur with severe injury and is more common on the left. Stomach and colon can pass into the chest but may not be immediately recognised because of the associated haemothorax or positive pressure ventilation preventing egress into the chest.

If the nasogastric tube turns up into the lower left chest, it indicates that the stomach is herniated.

AORTIC INJURY

The majority of patients with an aortic injury die at the scene of the accident.

Ninety-five per cent of aortic injuries occur at the aortic isthmus, i.e. at the level of the ligamentum arteriosum, just beyond the origin of the left subclavian artery. It is important to diagnose aortic injuries early because of the high mortality from delayed treatment.

Aortography, or more recently, CT aortography, is needed to establish or exclude the diagnosis of aortic rupture.

Aortography is indicated if the plain CXR shows the following signs:

- widened mediastinum
- effacement of the aortic arch contour and aortopulmonary window
- left pleural effusion
- left apical cap (haematoma)
- rightward deviation of the trachea
- deviation of the nasogastric tube in the oesophagus to the right
- depressed left main bronchus
- widening of the paraspinal stripe in the absence of a vertebral fracture.

The widened mediastinum is a non-specific, often subjective finding, and may be even projectional. Although it leads to many aortograms and CT aortograms (false positive finding), the actual detection of an aortic injury is life-saving.

CARDIAC INJURY

The right ventricle lies in the immediate retrosternal position and in a vulnerable position for penetrating and blunt injuries. Common cardiac injuries include myocardial contusion, haemopericardium and pneumopericardium. More severe injuries are coronary artery occlusion/laceration, myocardial infarction and pericardial tamponade.

If cardiac injury is suspected, then CT scanning, ECG and echocardiography will be necessary.

OESOPHAGEAL INJURY

An oesophageal tear is a rare injury after trauma. One mechanism is due to the sudden increase in intra-oesophageal pressure from the refluxing gastric contents. This causes a tear in the left posterolateral wall of the distal oesophagus, similar to the Boerhaave syndrome.

An oesophageal tear has the potential to cause mediastinitis if not detected. An oesophagogram with non-ionic contrast media or a CT scan will be necessary to make the diagnosis. Indirect signs are pneumomediastinum, left pneumothorax and pleural effusion.

The 'V sign of Naclerio' is an occasional sign that indicates an oesophageal tear. The air along the diaphragm (horizontal) and the para-oesophageal air (vertical) form a 'V'.

TRACHEOBRONCHIAL RUPTURE

In severe injuries, tears of the tracheal or bronchial wall can cause pneumomediastinum, subcutaneous emphysema and pneumothorax. The pneumothorax may persist despite tube drainage and this should alert the clinician to this possible injury. The tear most commonly occurs in the bronchus intermedius of the right lung. Complete rupture of a main bronchus can produce the 'fallen lung' sign.

TABLE 8.1	CXR review
Questions to be asked following review of the trauma CXR	
• Are there any subtle signs of a pneumothorax?	
• Are there any subtle signs of a pneumomediastinum?	
• Could a left pleural effusion be masking a diaphragmatic rupture?	
• Are there any signs of an aortic injury?	
• Are lateral views of the sternum or thoracic spine required?	

TABLE 8.2	Late complications of trauma
• Delayed aortic pseudoaneurysm/aortic rupture	
• Bowel herniated through a diaphragmatic rupture can obstruct	
• Bronchostenosis	
• ARDS	
• Fat embolism syndrome	
• Pulmonary hernia through disrupted ribs and intercostal muscles	
• Intrathoracic splenosis	
• Chylothorax (lymphatic duct tear)	
• Iatrogenic injuries from monitoring and life-support devices.	

OTHER CONDITIONS

- Non-accidental injury in children. Multiple rib fractures may indicate child abuse. Rickets and osteogenesis imperfecta need to be excluded.

- Cough fractures. Post-tussive fractures are insufficiency fractures in older osteoporotic patients. These are most common in the 4th to 9th ribs at the anterior axillary line. Because of the associated pleuritic pain, they can clinically mimic pulmonary emboli.

FURTHER READING

Schnyder P, Wintermark M, Baert AL. *Radiology of blunt trauma of the chest* (Berlin: Springer), 2000.

Chest X-ray <www.chestx-ray.com/lectures/ABCTrauma/BluntChestTr.html>

CHAPTER 9

MONITORING AND SUPPORT DEVICES—LINES, TUBES AND CATHETERS

INTRODUCTION

A disciplined approach to reviewing all parts of the chest X-ray is important. When lines, tubes or catheters have been inserted, the nature and location of all the support and/or monitoring devices are necessary observations in interpreting the chest X-ray. The lines, tubes or catheters have a radiopaque stripe to provide visibility on the radiograph.

A chest X-ray should be a routine image after insertion of a catheter to assure the correct position and identify complications. Obviously this is not necessary if the insertion has been under CT guidance.

ENDOTRACHEAL TUBE

An endotracheal tube is a tube inserted from the mouth or nose and into the trachea. It ensures patency of the airway and allows ventilation.

The lower end should be above the carina with the head and neck in the neutral position, i.e. tip in the mid trachea. Practically this places the lower end at the upper margin of the aortic arch.

During flexion and extension of the cervical spine, the lower end of the endotracheal tube will vary in position by up to 4 cm.

With neck flexion, the tip moves inferiorly, and with extension it moves superiorly. Any 2 cm excursion and carina movement on respiration can be safely accommodated.

If the endotracheal tube position is too high, the inflatable cuff has potential to damage the vocal cords or produce a neuropraxia of the internal laryngeal nerve. Also there is potential for accidental extubation with neck movement during patient transfers.

If intubation is too far, the endotracheal tube is more likely to enter the right mainstem bronchus because of the reduced angle on the right (see bronchial anatomy, Fig. 2.2 on page 13). This can cause complete collapse of the left lung and over distension of the right lung (or a complicating pneumothorax). Intubation beyond the main right bronchus, i.e. into the intermediate bronchus, can cause collapse of the right upper lobe as well, due to the early origin of the right upper lobe bronchus (see Fig. 2.1 on page 12).

Over distension of the endotracheal tube cuff will damage the tracheal wall cartilage and later may cause tracheomalacia or a stenosis.

A double lumen endotracheal tube is sometimes used for differential ventilation of the two lungs.

If there has been an unrecognised pharyngo-oesophageal intubation, a dilated oesophagus and stomach with small volume lungs will be observed.

Patients undergoing ventilation have an increased risk of pneumothorax due to high airway pressures, gas trapping and diseased lungs. Gas trapping may be due to inadequate expiratory time in the presence of COPD (volutrauma).

The high airway pressures may be due to stiff lungs, atelectasis, posture end-expiratory pressure, right mainstem bronchus intubation and manual over inflation.

The development of a tension pneumothorax may be preceded by the appearance of interstitial cysts or pulmonary interstitial emphysema (PIE).

A tension pneumothorax on mechanical ventilation may be rapidly fatal and requires immediate tube drainage.

TRACHEOSTOMY TUBES

Tracheostomy tubes may be used for long-term intubation or to bypass acute upper airway obstruction. Flexion and extension of the neck do not affect the position of the tracheostomy tube. As with the endotracheal tube, the cuff should not distend the tracheal wall.

NASOGASTRIC TUBES

Ideally, the tube should pass down the oesophagus so that the tip lies below the left hemidiaphragm in the stomach.

Incorrect positioning may show the tube tip lying above the gastro-oesophageal junction, coiled in the pharynx or passing into the tracheobronchial tree.

The anatomical shape of the stomach (well shown on CT scanning) is that the fundus lies posteriorly and the antrum anteriorly. Therefore if gastric fluid needs to be suctioned, the tip should be in the fundus. If air needs to be suctioned this is best done if the tip is in the antrum in a supine patient.

FEEDING TUBES

As with nasogastric tubes, the feeding tube should pass down the oesophagus. Under some circumstances, for example, gastroparesis, the tip may need to be in the distal duodenum to facilitate feeding and prevent gastro-oesophageal reflux and aspiration.

CENTRAL VENOUS CATHETER

There are three types of central venous devices: external central catheter, peripherally inserted central catheter (PICC) and subcutaneously implanted venous access devices.

The central venous catheter allows venous access, venous infusions and measurement of intravascular pressures (central venous pressure).

Central venous catheters are usually placed either through a subclavian or internal jugular vein approach. The optimal catheter tip position is in the superior vena cava.

Previously, the ideal catheter position was higher due to the concern over vessel perforation causing a haemopericardium. The catheter tip was therefore deliberately positioned above the level of the pericardial reflection. Nowadays with the softer polyurethane catheters, the tip is placed closer to the cavo-atrial junctions. However, a catheter tip advanced too far and positioned in the right atrium is associated with an increased risk of cardiac perforation, arrhythmias and marantic endocarditis; particularly, the larger diameter stiffer catheters used for dialysis e.g. Vas Cath. Similarly a left subclavian Vas Cath with the tip abutting the lateral wall of the SVC has the potential to erode.

Peripherally inserted central catheters (PICC) are placed via arm veins, commonly antecubital veins, and are useful for long-term

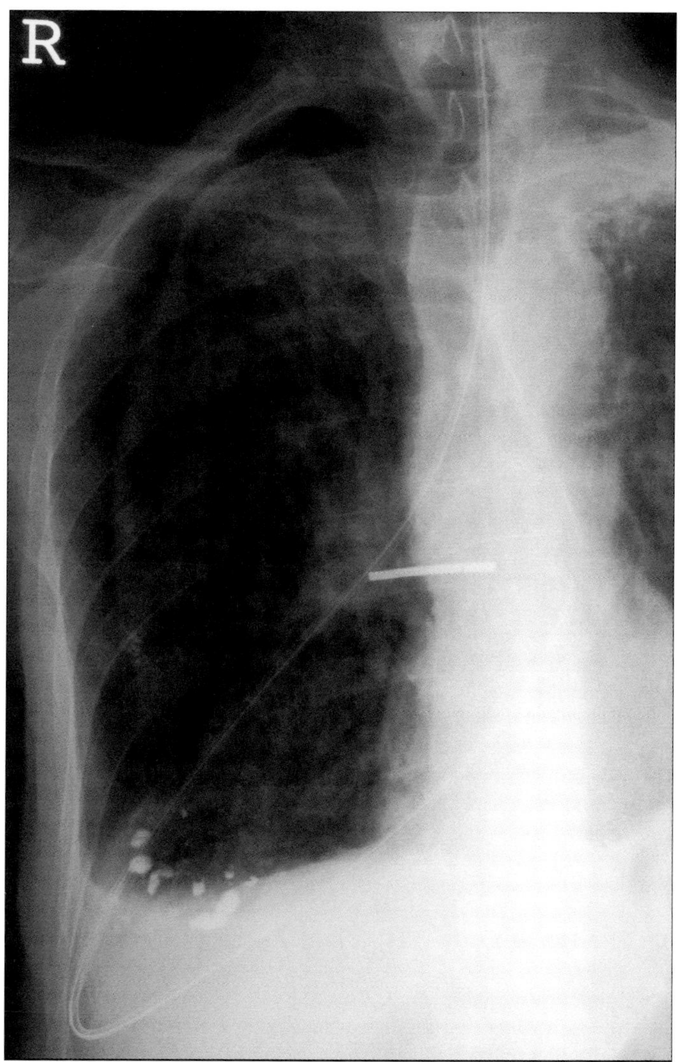

Fig. 9.1 Misplaced nasogastric tube

The nasogastric tube has passed down the tracheobronchial airway and penetrated the right lung, causing a pneumothorax.

There appears to be aspirated barium at the right lung base from a previous study.

access. They have a thin calibre and are flexible. The Groshong (Bard trademark) catheter has a valve near its rounded tip. This valve allows fluid infusion and blood aspiration. When not in use, the valve remains closed and restricts air embolism and blood backflow.

Hickman catheters are most often used for administration of chemotherapy and withdrawal of blood for chemotherapy. They are made of silastic (a silicone elastomere) and either double lumen or triple lumen varieties are available. They are tunnelled subcutaneously before being inserted into the access vein. The Dacron cuff needs to lie subcutaneously and forms a physical barrier as it adheres to the tissues. They are inserted for prolonged chemotherapy or TPN and have a lower incidence of infection.

'Vas Cath' and 'Permacath' are large bore dual-lumen catheters for dialysis.

On initial needling to find the vessel (subclavian or low jugular vein) a pneumothorax may occur. Inadvertent puncture of the subclavian or carotid artery may result in an extrapleural haematoma.

IMPLANTABLE VASCULAR ACCESS DEVICES

Port-A-Cath, Vital-Port, PAS-Port and POWERPort are subcutaneously implanted access reservoirs with attached central catheters.

Both the port reservoir and the attached catheter lie subcutaneously. The catheter passes into the subclavian vein or the IJV and then to the SVC. They are particularly useful in oncology patients with poor venous access. The plastic-covered, subcutaneous reservoir is accessible with special port needles.

POWERPorts will allow high flow injections of contrast agents for progress CT scans necessary in oncology patients.

PULMONARY ARTERY CATHETER

Pulmonary artery catheters are used in haemodynamically unstable patients to measure pulmonary artery pressure and cardiac output. The right ventricular pressure can also be measured during passage of the catheter.

Access is usually via the subclavian or internal jugular vein and the balloon-tip is floated past the pulmonic valve to lie proximally within the right or left pulmonary artery, which is the normal resting position. A well-known model is the Swan–Ganz catheter.

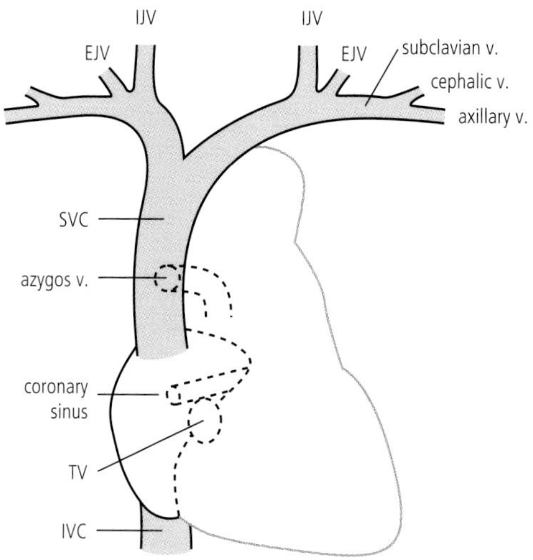

Fig. 9.2 Venous anatomy

The subclavian and internal jugular veins (IJV) join behind the clavicles to form the brachio-cephalic (or innominate) veins. The superior vena cava forms at the junction of the two brachio-cephalic veins behind the lower margin of the right first costal cartilage, at the level of the top of the aortic arch. The lower half of the SVC is invested by pericardium after being joined by the azygos vein.

When a 'wedge' measurement is required, the tip balloon is inflated and the catheter floats to a smaller artery. The measurement obtained is the pulmonary artery occlusion pressure (PAOP) that reflects the left atrial pressure and the left ventricular end-diastolic pressure (an indirect indicator of pre-load). This aids the differentiation between cardiogenic (hydrostatic) and non-cardiogenic (permeability) pulmonary oedema. The balloon should only be inflated during placement and pressure measurement and not left wedged in a small artery.

Complications are pulmonary infarction, haemorrhage and pseudoaneurysm formation. The serious complication is pulmonary artery rupture which can occur at the time of wedging or from rupture of a pseudoaneurysm. Pulmonary artery rupture has a mortality of 50%. Percutaneous transcatheter embolisation is the treatment of choice.

INTRA-AORTIC BALLOON PUMP (IABP)

Also known as the intra-aortic counterpulsation balloon catheter, it is used to improve cardiac function following cardiac surgery or in the treatment of cardiogenic shock. It supplements cardiac output by 25%.

By ECG coordination, it is inflated during diastole to increase myocardial perfusion, augmenting diastolic coronary artery perfusion and deflated in systole to decrease left ventricular work. Sometimes the sausage-shaped CO_2 carbon dioxide inflated balloon can be seen on the CXR if taken during diastole. A small radiopaque marker is present at the tip and ideally should be below the superior contour of the aortic knuckle, i.e. just distal to the left subclavian artery. If too low the counter pulsation is less effective. Introduced through the femoral artery, aortic wall dissection is a serious complication.

VENTRICULAR ASSIST DEVICE

This device is commonly surgically implanted in the left upper quadrant to relieve intractable congestive heart failure in patients awaiting transplantation.

PLEURAL DRAINAGE TUBES

These tubes are placed to remove air or fluid from the pleural space. They are either a larger thoracostomy tube or a smaller pigtail catheter.

To drain pleural fluid, the tube should be positioned in a gravity dependent position, i.e. in a supine patient in the posteroinferior chest. To drain a pneumothorax, the optimal position is the tip in the anterosuperior chest. After trauma, the pleural tube is placed from a subaxillary entry site to course posteriorly to the apex to drain air and blood.

Radiologic guidance is necessary where there have been failed non-guided attempts or where there is loculated pleural air or fluid collections.

Complications of intercostal tube drainage include bleeding from intercostal artery laceration. Laceration of the liver, spleen and stomach can occur due to perforation through the diaphragm. If the tube passes through the lung (pulmonary laceration) it can lead to further complications of haematoma and bronchopleural fistula. CT scanning is more accurate than the CXR if the chest tube is considered malpositioned, e.g. intrafissural.

If a pleural tube side-hole is in the chest wall, it could lead to subcutaneous emphysema or empyema necessitans (see Special effusions, Chapter 6). The side-hole is marked by the interruption of the radiopaque identification line and should lie medial to the inner rib margin.

CARDIAC PACEMAKERS AND AUTOMATIC IMPLANTABLE CARDIOVERTER-DEFIBRILLATION DEVICES

Pacemakers are used to correct conduction disorders. The pulse generator is an electronic battery powered device that is inserted subcutaneously. It is connected to lead wires which pass transvenously to the endocardium or myocardium. There are single chamber pacing (1 lead), dual chamber pacing (2 leads) and biventricular pacing (3 leads) pacemakers. With implantable cardioverter-defibrillators (ICD), the leads are larger and have a coiled spring appearance. The ICD electrode delivers an electrical pulse to the heart to interrupt life-threatening tachyarrhythmias.

Cardiac resynchronisation therapy is a treatment used in patients with terminal heart failure, e.g. significant left bundle branch block. It restores and coordinates effective ventricular contraction. Atrial synchronised biventricular pacing requires three leads to be inserted. One is in the right atrium, another in the right ventricle, and the third electrode wire is into a coronary vein (on the surface of the left ventricle) to pace the left ventricle. The atrial electrode is usually placed in the atrial appendage but may be placed nearby if the pacing threshold is favourable. Adhesions between the lead and the tricuspid valve leaflets can produce tricuspid insufficiency.

With other pacemakers, the leads may be placed by epicardially or via a subxiphoid approach rather than a transvenous route.

The chest X-ray inspection includes checking that the lead is not fractured. A common site of friction is between the clavicle and first rib (known as subclavian crush). By introducing the lead into the axillary or cephalic vein rather than the subclavian vein, or via the internal jugular vein route, this complication is avoided.

Magnetic resonance imaging is contra-indicated in patients with a pacemaker.

Other devices may be visible on the chest X-ray:

- sternal metallic cerclage wires
- pleural, pericardial and mediastinal drainage catheters
- metallic cardiac valves
- occlusion devices for intracardiac shunts
- loop recorders
- extracorporeal membrane oxygenation apparatus
- ventriculoperitoneal shunt tubes
- ECG leads
- implantable epicardial defibrillators with cardiac patches
- extrathoracic materials, e.g. oxygen tubing, electrocardiographic leads and buttons
- breast implants
- external pacemaker–defibrillator electrode plate
- plombage (used in the treatment of tuberculosis in the pre-antibiotic era)
- CABG clips and markers
- coronary artery stents
- SVC stent
- postoperative mediastinal and pericardial drains
- oesophageal stents and balloons
- temperature monitoring catheter in hypopharynx or oesophagus
- distal oesophageal pH probe
- embolisation coils
- ventricular assist devices.

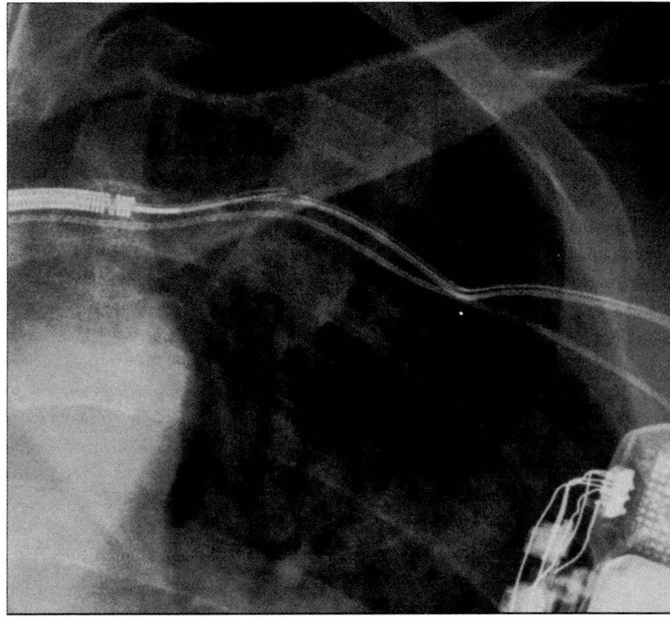

Fig. 9.3 Fractured lead

The defibrillator lead is shown to be fractured. It is difficult to know where the lead entered the subclavian vein but the fracture has occurred at a vulnerable position, i.e. in the costoclavicular canal.

TABLE 9.1 Complications table
Pleural drains
• lung laceration • cardiac perforation • vascular injury • re-expansion pulmonary oedema
Endotracheal tubes
• vocal cord injury • tracheal injury • atelectasis • oesophageal intubation • VILI, i.e. barotrauma and volutrauma
Nasogastric tube
• oesophageal perforation • transbronchial passage • lung perforation/pneumothorax
Intra-aortic balloon pump
• aortic dissection • leg ischaemia • renal or mesenteric ischaemia • cerebral infarct
Pulmonary artery catheter
• pulmonary infarct/haemorrhage • pulmonary artery pseudoaneurysm • coiling in right heart
Central venous catheter
• air embolism • malposition • pneumothorax • infusion into mediastinum • inadvertent arterial puncture/catheterisation • pinch-off syndrome • thrombosis
Pacemaker/Porta-A-Cath
• major vein thrombosis • PE • infection of device pocket • lead/catheter fracture

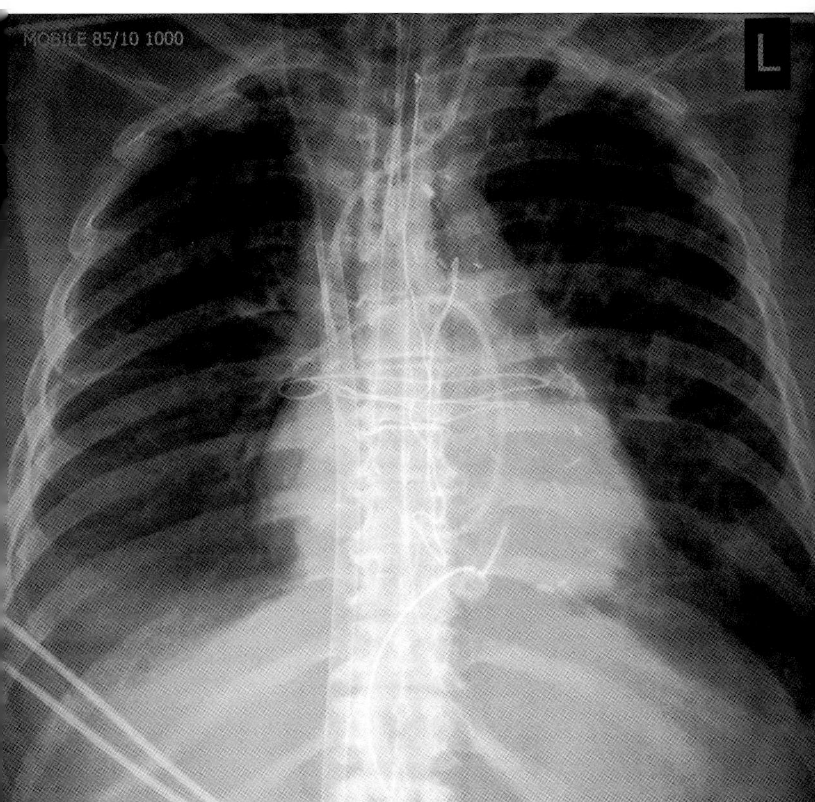

Fig. 9.4 Multiple devices

The radiograph shows an intensive care patient with a number of introduced tubes and catheters. The endotracheal tube is slightly low. The nasogastric tube does not pass beyond the lower oesophagus. The aortic balloon catheter (IACPB) has its tip in the distal arch and needs to be withdrawn. The right pulmonary artery catheter has been introduced from the right jugular vein. The ECMO tube passes into the SVC. Mediastinal drains are also present. The squiggly line opacities are due to radiopaque markers in the deliberately placed swabs in the sternal wound.

FURTHER READING

Hunter T. 'Medical Devices of the Chest'. *RadioGraphics* 2004; 24: 1725–46.

CHAPTER 10

PAEDIATRIC OVERVIEW

The interpretation of the paediatric chest radiograph requires knowledge of the congenital and pathological processes more likely to be seen in infants and children as well as an understanding of the special anatomical and physiological considerations.

SPECIAL ANATOMICAL CONSIDERATIONS

- The thymus is relatively large.
- The lung does not mature fully until 8 years of age. There are 20 million alveoli in the newborn lung and increasing to 300 million in the mature lung.
- The communications that allow for collateral airdrift in adults are much fewer in infants and young children. These are the pores of Kohn (intra-alveolar pores) and the channels of Lambert (bronchoalveolar channels).
- Up to the age of 15 years, there is symmetry in the right and left bronchial angles (compared to adult angles, p. 11). This explains why there is equal incidence of right- and left-sided aspiration of foreign bodies in children.
- The ductus arteriosus normally closes 1 to 2 days after birth. The ductus remains patent in hyaline membrane disease (HMD).
- The ductus venosus remains patent up to 4 days after birth and can be catheterised. The umbilical vein catheter will pass through it to enter the left (or middle) hepatic vein and enter the IVC. This catheter should pass straight upwards unlike the umbilical artery catheter which dips downwards to enter the internal iliac artery

and aorta. If the umbilical vein catheter changes course in the liver and does not pass upwards, it has entered the portal vein and could cause thrombosis.
- The ribs are more supple than in adults and less likely to fracture but there may be underlying lung contusion. Fractures without history of trauma should alert the radiologist to the possibility of non-accidental injury (NAI). Rib fractures, mid-clavicular fractures and humeral metaphyseal fractures may be evident on the chest X-ray in NAI.

OBSERVATIONAL CONSIDERATIONS

The rules of systematic inspection of the paediatric chest X-ray are the same as for adults (see Chapter 3) to ensure a thorough search. However, the observer must be aware of important differences in paediatric patients:
- The heart tends to be more globular in shape (many films are in the AP projection and there is not the full inspiration as expected in adults).
- The thymus is prominent (see sail sign, Appendix 2 and Fig. 2.7).
- In the left retrocardiac region, normal segmental air bronchograms may be seen below the left hilum.
- The growing bones look different from mature bones. Thorough CXR film interpretation requires inspection and knowledge of epiphyseal centres and metaphyseal plates.
- The volume of the lungs can be assessed by counting the ribs.

NEONATAL DISORDERS

Respiratory distress in the newborn needs to be recognised early, properly diagnosed and promptly managed. The salient points of the following respiratory diseases need to be known to distinguish them from neonatal pneumonia and the non-pulmonary causes of respiratory distress.

Transient tachypnoea

In the newborn this is also known as transient respiratory distress and retained fluid syndrome. It is a cause of self-limiting respiratory distress occurring in newborn full-term infants within 6 hours of birth, peaks at day 1, and resolves by the third day.

The foetal pulmonary fluid is usually cleared by the 'thoracic squeeze' during vaginal delivery. Delayed clearance by the capillaries and lymphatics leads to transient respiratory distress.

This condition is seen in babies born by caesarean section, sedated mothers and diabetic mothers. Its appearance may mimic congestive heart failure or a diffuse pneumonia. The lungs in transient tachypnoea are hyperinflated whereas in HMD the lungs are hypoinflated.

Meconium aspiration syndrome

This occurs as a result of meconium aspiration before or during birth; most commonly in post-mature neonates who have had intra-uterine foetal distress. The aspirated meconium causes small airways obstruction as well as a chemical pneumonitis. The chest X-ray shows hyperinflated lungs with coarse bilateral pulmonary infiltrates. The resultant respiratory distress can be complicated by a pneumothorax in a third of cases.

Amniotic fluid and gastric aspiration can also occur in the neonate and give rise to a similar radiographic appearance. However, resolution is much quicker.

Hyaline membrane disease

HMD, alternatively known as respiratory distress syndrome but better named as surfactant-deficient disease, is the most common cause of respiratory distress in the premature infant.

The premature type II pneumocytes are unable to produce sufficient surfactant which normally coats the alveolar surface, reduces surface tension and prevents end expiratory alveolar collapse. The non-compliant lungs have a low volume with diffuse granular opacities representing the collapsed alveoli. This reticulogranular appearance is seen in the mild to moderate cases, progressing to complete opacification of the lungs (with air bronchograms) in the more severe cases. Pleural effusions are uncommon.

Treatment of HMD includes synthetic surfactant and ventilation.

The mechanical ventilation of the stiff lungs in HMD can lead to barotrauma complications and bronchopulmonary dysplasia. The barotrauma complications include pulmonary interstitial emphysema, pneumothorax, pneumomediastinum and pneumopericardium.

Bronchopulmonary dysplasia

This chronic lung injury is a complication of prolonged ventilation, most frequently with HMD. It is thought to be due to a combination of oxygen toxicity (oxygen alveolopathy) and positive pressure ventilation (PPV). The initial phase is a permeability oedema (see 'leaky lung syndrome', Appendix 1) with a hazy density. Later, there are coarse reticular markings and cystic lucencies (bubbly lung) due to heterogeneous aeration of the lung parenchyma. Some alveolar groups overdistend, coalesce and form bubbles whereas others are collapsed.

Pulmonary interstitial emphysema

PIE is a complication of ventilation of premature infants with immature lungs. Air escapes from ruptured alveolar ducts into the interstitium, lymphatics and venous system.

Neonatal pneumonia

Although there are many possible infectious agents, β-haemolytic (group B) streptococcal pneumonia is the most common pneumonia seen in neonates. It can cause low volume lungs with a granular appearance, similar to HMD, but in contrast to HMD, often has associated pleural effusions.

INFANT AND CHILDHOOD DISORDERS

Paediatric pneumonia

In all age groups, viral infections are much more common than bacterial infections. The viral infections are common because immunity has not developed unlike adults. The parainfluenza viruses and respiratory syncytial virus are the main pathogens.

In school-aged children, although viral agents remain the most common cause of lower respiratory tract infections, the incidence of *Streptococcus pneumoniae* and *Mycoplasma pneumoniae* increases.

Foreign body aspiration

The presence of a foreign body needs to be considered in children who present with a cough or persisting pneumonia.

Asthma

As in adults, the commonest appearance is a normal radiograph. During an acute exacerbation, hyperinflation may be present. The indicators for the CXR are demonstration of any concomitant infection, possible complications (such as pneumomediastinum or pneumothorax) or asthma mimics (foreign body wheezing).

Chronic bronchial wall thickening may be seen due to mucosal oedema.

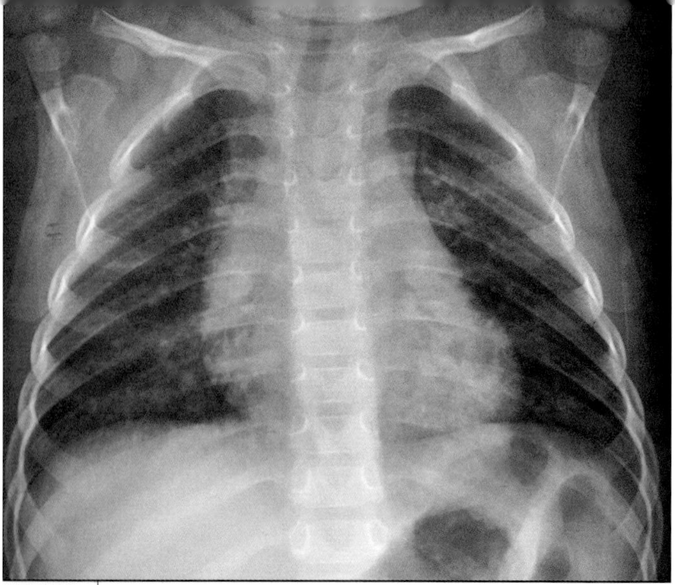

FIG 10.1a

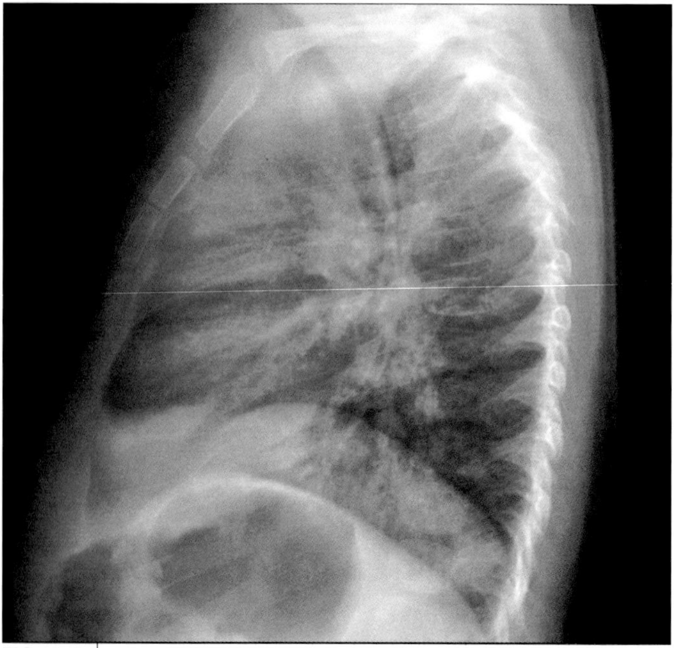

FIG 10.1b

Fig. 10.1 Viral bronchitis (a) frontal view; (b) lateral view

Streaky hazy shadowing is seen in both lungs, especially near the hila. These parahilar peribronchial opacities are a pattern seen with viral bronchitis and are due to peribronchial inflammation and oedema. A bacterial pneumonia is more likely to produce a peripheral area of consolidation.

CONGENITAL RESPIRATORY CONDITIONS

Congenital pulmonary hypoplasia is associated with hypoplasia of the ipsilateral pulmonary artery. It needs to be distinguished from Swyer–James syndrome that has an acquired hypoplastic lung following severe obliterative bronchiolitis. The hypoplastic Swyer–James lung shows considerable air trapping.

Cystic adenomatoid malformation is a hamartomatous lesion consisting of solid (dysplastic adenomatous tissue) and cystic elements. In the first few days of life, the cysts are fluid filled and then become air filled due to their bronchial communication. The radiographic appearances and the typing (types 1, 2 and 3) depend on the size of the cysts.

Congenital lobar emphysema is over-inflation of a lobe due to a developmental abnormality of the supplying bronchus. When the fluid clears, the affected lobe is hyperlucent and expanded. Most commonly affected is the left upper lobe, followed by the right middle lobe and the right upper lobe (see Fig. 10.3).

Diaphragmatic hernia can cause respiratory distress at birth. The most common type is the left posterolateral (Bochdalek type) hernia. There is herniation of the stomach, bowel and other organs into the chest. The ipsilateral lung is poorly aerated and hypoplastic with mediastinal shift.

Tracheo-oesophageal fistula is associated with oesophageal atresia and many other congenital abnormalities, e.g. VATER/VACTERL complex.

Bronchopulmonary sequestration (pulmonary sequestration) is detached from the normal lung, has no bronchial communication and is supplied by an anomalous systemic artery. They may be intralobar or extralobar in type. The intralobar type shares the same visceral pleura and has a draining pulmonary vein. Many of the intralobar sequestrations are probably acquired, rather than congenital, and due to chronic bronchial obstruction and infection.

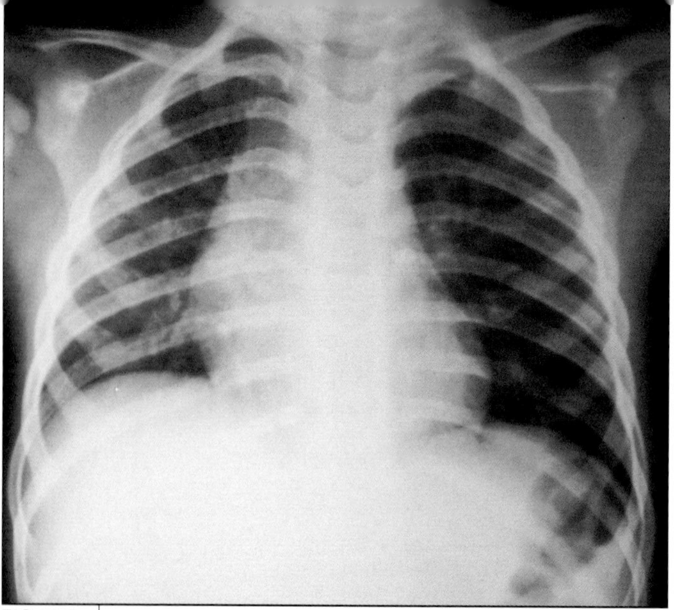

FIG 10.2a

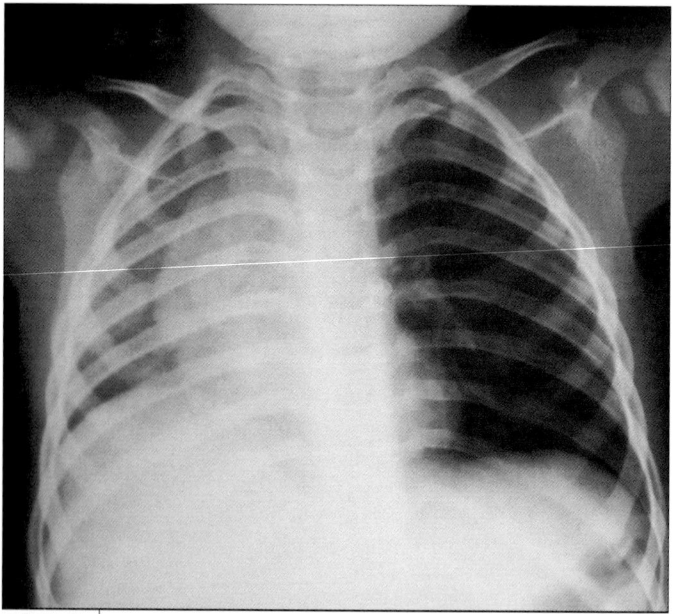

FIG 10.2b

Fig. 10.2 Inhaled foreign body (a) inspiration; (b) expiration

An 18-month-old child with acute onset of cough and dyspnoea. This is due to an inhaled foreign body (just visible) in the left main bronchus with hyperinflation of the left lung. This is exaggerated on the expiratory view due to air trapping, resulting in mediastinal shift to the right and depression of the left hemidiaphragm.

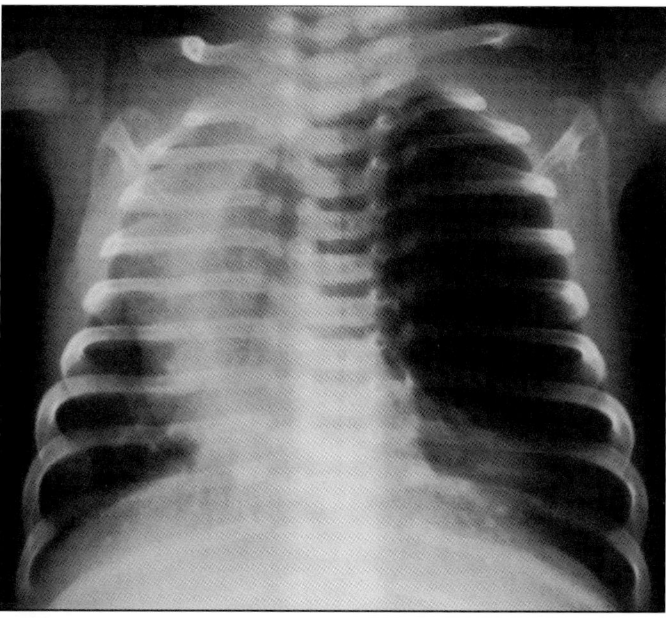

Fig. 10.3 Congenital lobar emphysema

There is hyperinflation of the left upper lobe with vessel paucity, herniation across the midline, mediastinal shift and left lower lobe compressive atelectasis. The left upper lobe is the most commonly involved lobe (45% of cases).

The extralobar sequestration is less frequent, enclosed in its own pleural membrane and drains into a systemic vein. The extralobar sequestration is always congenital.

The posterior basal segment is the most commonly involved. It appears radiographically as a homogeneous opacity ('persisting pneumonia') or a cystic mass.

It is surgically important that thoracic and upper abdominal aortography or CT angiogram is performed before surgery to identify the anomalous systemic artery which may arise from below the diaphragm.

A *bronchogenic cyst* is a type of foregut duplication cyst due to abnormal budding off the embryonic tracheobronchial tree. Many lie in the mediastinum near the carina but some are pulmonary.

Cystic fibrosis is a multisystem disease due to abnormal viscid secretions from the exocrine glands (mucoviscidosis). It is an autosomal recessive hereditary disease with no sex preponderance and is a common serious genetic disease in Caucasians, with an incidence of 1 in 2,000 live births. Although more vigilant treatment has improved outcome, without transplantation the life expectancy is about 30 years of age.

The thick tenacious mucus causes obstruction of the small airways followed by infection and inflammation. The radiographic findings are of scarred lungs which are hyperinflated. There is evidence of bronchiectasis, bronchial wall thickening and mucous plugging. The hila are prominent due to lymphadenopathy from chronic infection and, in longstanding disease, pulmonary artery dilatation due to PAH.

CONGENITAL HEART DISEASE

There are many congenital malformations of the heart and great vessels. These require intensive investigation with echocardiography, cardiac catheterisation, MRI and CT scanning. The CXR is performed to assess pulmonary vascularity, heart size, aortic position and for any unsuspected abnormalities.

Clinically, the child is either cyanosed or not.

Radiographically, the pulmonary vascularity is either increased (congested), normal or decreased. Often the CXR is normal.

Left-to-right shunts

The most common shunts are:

- Patent ductus arteriosus(PDA)

- Atrial septal defect (ASD)
- Ventricular septal defect (VSD)

Atrial septal defect, ventricular septal defect and patent ductus arteriosus produce left-to-right shunting. When the shunting is more than 2:1, there is cardiac enlargement, central pulmonary artery enlargement (prominent hila) and pulmonary plethora.

Right-to-left shunts (cyanotic heart disease)

The five common right-to-left shunts are:

- Tetralogy of Fallot (commonest)
- Transposition
- Truncus arteriosus
- Triscuspid atresia
- Total anomalous pulmonary venous return ('snowman' sign)

Tetralogy of Fallot

Fallot's tetralogy is the fourth most common congenital cardiac abnormality but the most common cyanotic heart defect. It is the most common cause of decreased pulmonary vascularity.

By definition it consists of:

- infundibular right ventricular outflow tract stenosis
- subaortic VSD
- overriding aorta
- right ventricular hypertrophy

In about half the cases, the CXR can have a normal appearance. However, the classic radiological sign is a boot-shaped heart (coeur en sabot) where the cardiac apex is pushed upwards and outwards by the right ventricular hypertrophy.

Because the pulmonary trunk is hypoplastic there is a prominent pulmonary bay, i.e. curved depression.

Oligaemia (decreased pulmonary vascularity) is seen in the lungs.

In 25% of patients, the aorta is right-sided. In 10%, there is in addition an atrial septal defect (pentalogy of Fallot).

Milder cases with smaller VSDs and less right ventricular outflow obstruction may present later in life and are sometimes referred to as 'pink tetralogy'.

Coarctation of the aorta

Dilatation of the aorta proximal and distal to the coarctation results in the characteristic 'figure 3' sign.

Rib notching is not seen until late childhood (see Fig. 3.1).

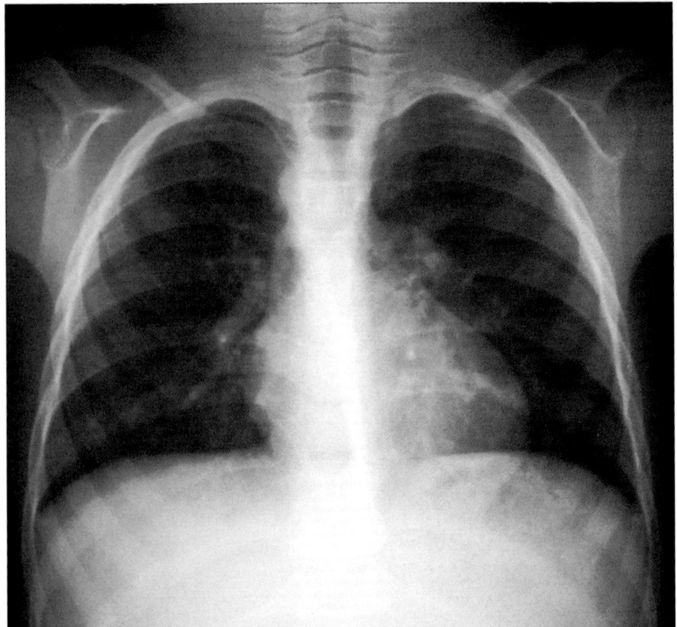

Fig. 10.4 Tetralogy of Fallot
The lungs are oligaemic. The heart shadow is tending towards a boot shape. Note that the aortic knuckle is on the right side of the trachea.

Total or partial anomalous pulmonary venous return (TAPVR)

Scimitar syndrome (congenital pulmonary venolobar syndrome)

The scimitar (Turkish sword) is a curved band density at the right lower zone representing an anomalous pulmonary vein draining into the IVC. This condition is a form of partial anomalous pulmonary venous drainage. It is associated with a small right lung with under-development of both the bronchial tree and vascular structures. Besides the hypoplastic right pulmonary artery, a branch of the aorta also supplies the right lung.

Truncus arteriosis septation anomalies

Anomalies of septation of the embryonic truncus arteriosus into the aorta and the pulmonary trunk are:

- Tetralogy of Fallot
- Truncus arteriosus
- Pulmonary atresia
- Transposition

Cardiac malposition

Normally, the cardiac apex lies to the left of the spine. Abnormal cardiac positions are seen in dextrocardia, dextroversion and the heterotaxia syndromes.

FURTHER READING

WEB PAGES

There are several teaching files and other resources online:

<http://www.chestx-ray.com>
<http://www.eurorad.org>—go to Chest Imaging
<http://www.lsbu.ac.uk/dirt/museum/
<http://www.mypacs.net>
<http://www.med.wayne.edu/diagRadiology>—go to Education
<http://www.uhrad.com>—go to the section on Body Imaging
<http://www.auntminnie.com>—go to Reference and then Thoracic Radiology
<http://www.brighamrad.harvard.edu/fire>
<http://www.mds.qmw.ac.uk/radiology/>
<http://www.ctisus.org>
<http://www.meddean.luc.edu/lumen/MedEd/medicine/pulmonar/cxr/cxr.htm>
<http://www.radport.com/teach.html>
<http://www.radiology.co.uk/srs-x/>
<http://www.med-ed.virginia.edu/courses/rad/cxr/index.html>
<http://www.radiologyeducation.org>
<http://www.learningradiology.com>

BIBLIOGRAPHY

Burgener F, Kormano M. Differential diagnosis in chest x-rays. Stuttgart: Thieme, 1997.

Collins CD, Lopez A, Mathie A, Wood V, Jackson JE, Roddie ME. 'Quantification of pneumothorax size on chest radiographs using interpleural distances'. *AJR* 1995; 165:1127.

Collins J, Stern E. *Chest radiology: The essentials*. 2nd edn. Baltimore: Lippincott Williams & Wilkins, 2007.

DeLacey G, Morley S, Berman L. *The chest X-ray: A survival guide*. Philadelphia: Saunders Elsevier, 2008.

Donnelly LF. *Fundamentals of paediatric radiology*. Philadelphia: WB Saunders, 2001.

Figley MM, Gerdes AJ, Ricketts HJ. 'Radiographic aspects of pulmonary embolism'. *Semin Roentgenol* 1967;2:389–405.

Fraser R, Pare JAP, Pare PD et al. *Diagnosis of diseases of the chest*. 3rd edn. Philadelphia: WB Saunders Co., 1998.

Gurney JW, Winer-Muram HT. et al. *Diagnostic imaging – chest*. Salt Lake City: Amirys, 2006.

Hansell DM, Armstrong P, Lynch DA, McAdams HP. *Imaging of diseases of the chest*. 3rd edn. London: Elsevier Mosby 2005.

Hofer M, Abanador N, Rattunde H, Zentai C, Kamper L. *The Chest X-ray: A systematic teaching atlas*. Stuttgart: Thieme, 2007.

Kazerooni EA and Gross B. *Cardiopulmonary Imaging*. Philadelphia: Lippincott Williams & Wilkins, 2003.

Lange S and Walsh G. *Radiology of chest diseases*. 3rd edn. Stuttgart: Thieme, 2005.

McLoud TC. *Thoracic radiology: The requisites*. St Louis: Mosby, 1998.

Matsushima T, Eguchi K, Kuwabara M. *Diseases of the chest: Imaging diagnosis based on pattern classification*. Stuttgart: Thieme, 2002.

Mergo PJ. *Imaging of the chest: A teaching file*. Baltimore: Lippincott Williams & Wilkins, 2002.

Muller NL and Silva CIS. *Imaging of the chest*. Philadelphia: Saunders Elsevier, 2008.

Parker MS, Rosado-de-Christenson ML, Abbott GF. *Teaching atlas of chest imaging*. Stuttgart: Thieme, 2005.

Schnyder P, Wintermark M, Baert AL. *Radiology of blunt trauma of the chest* (Berlin: Springer), 2000.

Sutton D, ed. *Textbook of radiology and imaging*. 7th edn. Edinburgh: Churchill Livingstone.

Webb WR and Higgins CB. *Thoracic imaging*. Philadelphia: Lippincott Williams & Wilkins, 2005.

Wright F. *Radiology of the chest and related conditions*. London: Taylor and Francis, 2002.

GLOSSARY REFERENCES

Hansell DM. 'Fleischner Society: Glossary of terms for thoracic imaging'. *Radiology* March 2008; 246(3): 697–722.

Webb RW, Muller NL, Naidich DP. 'Illustrated glossary in high-resolution computed tomography terms'. In: *High resolution CT of the lung*. 3rd edn. Baltimore: Lippincott Williams & Wilkins, 2001: 599–618.

APPENDIX 1

SYNDROMES RELEVANT TO CHEST RADIOLOGY

The term syndrome derives from the Greek and literally means 'run together'. So syndrome refers to the association of several signs and symptoms. A specific disease may or may not be identified as the underlying cause.

A list of eponymous and non-eponymous syndromes is provided to alert the reader to the extent of conditions involving the chest. Some are congenital, others are acquired.

Acquired immunodeficiency syndrome (AIDS) Human immunodeficiency virus (HIV) infection and a $CD4^+$ T lymphocyte count < 200/μL.

Acute chest syndrome General term used in patients with sickle-cell haemoglobinopathy who develop fever and chest symptoms and signs; due to either pneumonia or pulmonary infarction.

An alternative explanation is that there are rib infarcts with secondary splinting and lung atelectasis.

Acute coronary syndrome An umbrella term for types of acute myocardial ischaemia including myocardial infarction and unstable angina. The commonest cause is disruption of an atherosclerotic plaque in a coronary artery, producing chest pain.

Adult respiratory distress syndrome (ARDS) An advanced form of increased permeability (non-cardiogenic) pulmonary oedema. The lung injury is the diffuse alveolar damage, hyaline membrane formation and cellular infiltration. There are exudative, proliferative and fibrotic phases. Radiographically there are diffuse lung parenchymal opacities in low volume lungs. Clinically there is severe hypoxaemia and reduced lung compliance. Also known as 'shock lung', 'stiff lung' and Da Nang syndrome.

Air-leak syndrome Uncommon late complication in haemopoeitic stem cell recipients with chronic graft-versus-host disease and related bronchiolitis obliterans. Pneumomediastinum, pneumothorax, interstitial emphysema or subcutaneous emphysema may occur.

Aspiration syndromes (see Chapter 4) Aspiration of different substances into the airways and lungs can have a range of consequences depending on the volume and type of material, e.g. inert, irritant or infectious.

Asplenia syndrome (double right-sideness). Absent spleen and bilateral trilobed lungs. Double SVC and left IVC. Immunosuppressed for encapsulated bacteria and therefore susceptible to sepsis. Also known as Ivemark syndrome (see Heterotaxia syndrome).

Behçet's disease Chronic relapsing vasculitis secondary to immune complex deposition; also known as Hughes–Stovin syndrome.

Birt–Hogg–Dubé syndrome Autosomal dominant disease with thin-walled subpleural basal cysts. One cause of familial spontaneous pneumothorax.

Blesovsky syndrome Round atelectasis or folded lung that resembles a mass; can be a consequence of asbestos exposure.

Boerhaave syndrome Severe vomiting can cause a tear in the oesophageal wall leading to acute mediastinitis. The tear is usually in the left posterolateral wall of the distal oesophagus where muscle and extramural support are deficient. A similar tear can occur in trauma.

Caplan syndrome Pulmonary nodules developing in coal miners with rheumatoid arthritis.

Carney triad Multiple pulmonary chrondromas, gastric leiomyoblastoma and phaeochromacytoma.

Churg–Strauss syndrome Small vessel vasculitis in patients with asthma and peripheral eosinophilia; also called allergic granulomatosis and angiitis, and allergic granulomatosis.

Ciliary dyskinesia syndrome Impaired mucociliary clearance causes recurrent upper and lower respiratory tract infections. Also known as immobile (immotile) ciliary syndrome.

Combined pulmonary fibrosis and emphysema (CPFE) Characterised by both emphysema of the upper zones and diffuse parenchymal lung disease with fibrosis (UIP) in the lower zones. Subnormal spirometry, gas exchange impairment and pulmonary hypertension produce a poor survival. It is postulated that smoking is the predominant risk factor for both entities.

Congenital pulmonary venolobar syndrome A form of partial anomalous pulmonary venous return. Hypoplastic right lung with a prominent pulmonary vein (scimitar sign) draining into the inferior vena cava. Also known as the hypogenetic lung syndrome and scimitar syndrome.

CREST syndrome (see CREST acronym) Less severe skin involvement than classic systemic sclerosis (scleroderma).

Doege–Potter syndrome Symptomatic hypoglycaemia associated with malignant neoplasms and solitary fibrous tumour of the pleura.

Dressler syndrome Fever, pleuritis, pneumonitis and pericarditis occurring a few days or weeks after myocardial infarction.

A similar syndrome occurs after cardiac surgery (post-pericardiotomy syndrome) or chest trauma (post-cardiac injury syndrome).

Dyskinetic cilia syndrome See Ciliary dyskinesia syndrome.

Ebstein anomaly Downward displacement of the tricuspid valve into the right ventricle and associated great enlargement of the right atrium.

Ehlos–Danlos syndrome Underlying defect in the elastic tissue; can be complicated by an aortic aneurysm.

Eisenmenger syndrome or **Eisenmenger reaction** Severe pulmonary arterial hypertension due to a left-to-right shunt. Eventually the pulmonary artery pressures increase so much as to cause a reversal of the blood flow so that deoxygenated blood from the right heart passes to the left heart and then body causing cyanosis.

Fallot tetralogy The primary changes are infundibular stenosis and a high ventricular septal defect. Overriding of the aorta and right ventricular hypertrophy are the secondary structural defects.

Fat embolism syndrome Harmful effects of fat embolism on the lungs (DAD and ARDS) and other organs. Although fat embolism from long bone fractures is common, it only rarely leads to fat embolism syndrome. Early immobilisation of fractures can reduce fat embolism. Non-traumatic fat embolism is due to circulating lipids and mobilised fat. (See the causes of fat embolism syndrome, Appendix 3).

Goodpasture syndrome One of the pulmonary–renal syndromes manifesting as diffuse pulmonary haemorrhage and glomerulonephritis.

Hamman–Rich syndrome Acute interstitial pneumonia which is a rapidly progressive form of lung injury representing an idiopathic form of diffuse alveolar damage (DAD) and/or acute respiratory distress syndrome (ARDS).

Hantavirus pulmonary syndrome Infection with the hantavirus causes severe damage to pulmonary capillary endothelium with consequential pulmonary oedema of the increased permeability type.

Hepatopulmonary syndrome A complication of end-stage liver disease without intrinsic lung disease. Functional arteriovenous shunting in the lungs causes arterial hypoxaemia.

Hereditary haemorrhagic telangiectasia Also known as Rendu–Osler–Weber or Osler–Weber–Rendu syndrome. In about 10% of these patients arteriovenous malformations occur in the lungs.

Heterotaxia syndrome Also known as situs ambiguous, and cardiosplenic syndromes. Disturbance of the normal orderly left-right asymmetry in the positions of the thoracic and abdominal organs. Two subtypes are the Asplenia (Ivemark) syndrome and the Polysplenia syndrome. Very high incidence of congenital heart disease.

Horner syndrome Eye signs. Local ipsilateral destruction of the sympathetic chain by a Pancoast tumour.

Hughes–Stovin syndrome A rare variant of Behçet's disease in that patients only exhibit some features.

Hypereosinophilic syndrome Multi-organ infiltration by eosinophils. Blood, BAL and tissue eosinophilia but no cause (such as parasites, drugs or allergies) is recognised. Cardiac involvement in 75% of patients. Pulmonary and pleural involvement in 40%. Cardiomegaly, pulmonary oedema, transient consolidation, GGO and pleural effusions can occur.

Hypertrophic pulmonary osteoarthropathy. Characterised by digital clubbing, polyarthralgia and periostitis. Often a paraneoplastic syndrome because lung cancer is the most common cause. Secondary hypertrophic osteopathy is a better term as there are nonpulmonary causes such as inflammatory bowel disease and congenital cardiac anomalies. See Appendix 3.

Hypogenetic lung syndrome Hypoplastic right lung with anomalous pulmonary vein draining into the inferior vena cava. Also known as congenital pulmonary venolobar syndrome and scimitar syndrome (see scimitar sign).

Idiopathic pulmonary fibrosis Gradual onset of dyspnoea, fine crackles on auscultation and digital clubbing. The early phase shows predominantly basal reticular shadowing and progresses to honeycombing with lower zone volume loss. Histologically is usually UIP.

Immune reconstitution inflammatory syndrome or **immune restoration syndrome**. HIV-infected patients may show a transient clinical decline to latent opportunistic infection and an exuberant inflammatory response as their immune system recovers when antiretroviral therapy is begun.

Kartagener syndrome Situs inversus (dextrocardia), bronchiectasis and sinusitis.

Klippel–Trenauney–Weber syndrome Numerous arteriovenous malformations which can involve the chest wall.

Lady Windermere syndrome Non-tuberculous mycobacterial infection occurring in patients without underlying lung disease. These patients are usually elderly females who have an irritating chronic cough. A 'tree-in-bud' appearance is seen on HRCT, mainly occurring in the right middle lobe and lingular segment.

Leaky lung syndrome The initial oedematous phase of bronchopulmonary dysplasia which is a complication of ventilated neonates. Fluid leaks across the damaged basement membrane of the capillaries (permeability pulmonary oedema) into the interstitium as in the early phase of ARDS/acute lung injury.

Lemierre syndrome Parapharyngeal infection causing suppurative thrombophlebitis of the internal jugular vein. It may cause septic pulmonary emboli.

Loeffler syndrome Patchy migratory infiltrates on CXR due to an allergic reaction to parasitic infiltration of lungs.

MacLeod syndrome Acquired hypoplasia of one lung secondary to infantile obliterative bronchiolitis; consequential small pulmonary artery and bronchiectasis. Also known as Swyer–James syndrome.

Marfan syndrome Connective disease disorder; predisposed to aortic aneurysms and dissections.

Meconium aspiration syndrome Occurs when an infant aspirates meconium into the lungs before or during delivery. The meconium can block the airways, cause a chemical pneumonitis and reduce gas exchange.

Meigs syndrome Non-neoplastic pleural effusion and ascites associated with a benign ovarian tumour (a malignant ovarian tumour needs to be excluded). Also known as Meigs–Salmon syndrome.

Mendelson syndrome Chronic or recurrent collapse of the right middle lobe and/or lingula. It can be due to either extraluminal or intraluminal bronchial obstruction, but also may develop without identifiable obstruction where the lobar bronchus is patent. Aspiration of gastric juice causing a chemical pneumonitis.

Middle lobe syndrome Chronic or recurrent collapse of the right middle lobe and/or lingula. It can be due to either extraluminal or intraluminal bronchial obstruction, but also may develop without identifiable obstruction where the lobar bronchus is patent. Bronchiectasis may be present in the collapsed lobe. TB is a common cause.

Mounier–Kuhn syndrome Tracheobronchomegaly.

Organic dust toxic syndrome Exposure to organic dusts can cause an influenza-like symptom complex.

Paget–Schrotter syndrome Thrombosis of the subclavian vein due to compression between the clavicle and first rib ('effort thrombosis').

Pancoast syndrome Symptom complex of pain in the shoulder or arm from an apical tumour invading the brachial plexus and sympathetic chain (unilateral Horner syndrome).

Paraneoplastic syndromes Are defined as clinical syndromes involving non-metastatic systemic effects that accompany malignant disease. The symptoms occur remotely from the tumour itself and are due to substances produced by the tumour.

Pickwickian syndrome Morbidly obese with alveolar hypoventilation and pulmonary hypertension.

Pinch-off syndrome Also known as the 'subclavian crush'. The compression of the central venous catheter between the clavicle and first rib. This can lead to catheter or electrode lead fracture. This narrow space is also responsible for the thoracic outlet syndrome and Schrotter–Paget syndrome.

Poland syndrome Congenital defect of the pectoral muscle.

Polysplenia syndrome (double left-sideness) Multiple spleens and bilateral bilobed lungs. Double SVC and absent infrahepatic IVC. Dilated azygos vein. (See Heterotaxia syndrome).

Post-thoracotomy pain syndrome Chronic myofascial pain that occurs in the general area of the incision and persists at least two months after the thoracotomy.

Pseudo-mitral stenosis syndrome Clinically similar to severe mitral stenosis but due to stenosis of the proximal pulmonary veins in fibrosing mediastinitis.

Rendu–Osler–Weber syndrome Hereditary haemorrhagic telangiectasia with multiple arteriovenous malformations.

Respiratory distress syndrome (neonatal) Also known as hyaline membrane disease is due to deficient surfactant, most commonly affecting premature infants (see hyaline membrane disease, Chapter 10).

Riley–Day syndrome Hereditary neurological disease with dysplasia and recurrent episodes of aspiration bronchopneumonia; consequential bronchiectasis.

SAPHO syndrome—synovitis, acne, pustulosis, hyperosteitis and osteotis. The upper chest wall is involved, i.e. clavicles, first ribs and sternum as well as the sternoclavicular and manubriosternal joints.

Severe acute respiratory syndrome (SARS) Influenza-like infection caused by a coronavirus.

Scimitar syndrome Also known as congenital pulmonary venolobar syndrome and hypogenetic lung syndrome.

Sjögren syndrome Polyarthritis with dry mucous membranes; also known as sicca syndrome.

Superior vena cava syndrome Occlusion of the SVC either by thrombus or tumour or fibrosing mediastinitis. The patient will present with a congested and oedematous face and upper limbs.

Swyer–James syndrome See MacLeod syndrome.

Thoracic outlet syndrome Impingement of the brachial plexus, sublcavian artery or subclavian vein due to compression between the clavicle and first rib, or due to congenital fibromuscular band off the C7 transverse process (see Paget–Schrotter syndrome).

Tropical eosinophilia Episodic cough and wheezing, high blood eosinophilia and diffuse reticulonodular infiltrates on the chest radiograph.

Twiddler syndrome Rotation of a chest wall pacemaker which causes dislodgement of the electrodes, resulting in pacemaker malfunction.

Vanishing lung syndrome Markedly progressive emphysema with giant bullae in young men who are usually smokers.

Wet lung syndrome Also known as transient tachypnoea of the newborn, transient respiratory distress of the newborn, and retained fluid syndrome. This is a self-limiting cause of respiratory distress due to uncleared fetal pulmonary fluid.

Williams–Campbell syndrome Tracheobronchomalacia.

Wilson–Mikity syndrome A form of pulmonary dysmaturity in premature neonates which differs from bronchopulmonary dysplasia in that there is no history of hyaline membrane disease, prolonged oxygen therapy or mechanical ventilation.

Yellow nail syndrome A triad of yellow nails, pleural effusion and primary lymphoedema. Other respiratory manifestations include recurrent bronchitis, pneumonia, pleurisy, bronchiectasis and sinusitis.

Young syndrome A rare syndrome with sinopulmonary infection and bronchiectasis. It clinically resembles ciliary dyskinesia syndrome but ciliary function is normal and infertility is due to obstructive azoospermia.

APPENDIX 2

SIGNS IN THORACIC RADIOLOGY

A 'sign' in radiology refers to an abnormal radiological finding that suggests a specific disease process or possible group of disorders. The sign facilitates the interpretation by providing a clue. A 'pattern' refers to a collection of radiological findings.

The basic signs in chest radiology are:

- air bronchogram
- atelectasis
- bronchial wall thickening
- calcification
- cavitation
- consolidation
- ground-glass opacity
- mass/nodule
- reticular shadowing

The following signs are used in thoracic radiology. Because of overlap and to help with understanding of disease processes, CT signs have been included for completeness.

acinar pattern A collection of poorly defined or partly confluent opacities. They are 4–8 mm in diameter and together produce an inhomogeneous shadow. Similar terms are rosette pattern and acinose pattern (used specifically for endobronchial spread of tuberculosis).

air bronchogram sign The bronchus is visible as an air-filled structure surrounded by consolidated or collapsed lung. The most common causes are pneumonia and alveolar pulmonary oedema. When associated with collapse, its presence implies that the bronchus is not obstructed at its origin. Pulmonary lymphoma and alveolar cell carcinoma are tumours that can have a characteristic air bronchogram sign. Severe interstitial fibrosis and radiation fibrosis can produce air bronchograms due to the airless lung. Air bronchograms may be visible in the left retrocardiac region of normal children from the segmental bronchi (see B6 bronchus sign).

air crescent (meniscus) sign A radiolucent crescent becomes apparent at the periphery of a pulmonary mass lesion or when an area of pneumonia undergoes necrosis and cavitates. It most commonly occurs with an intracavitary fungus ball but can also be seen in hydatid cyst, lung abscess, haematoma and tumours.

air-fluid level Indicates bronchial communication if seen within a pulmonary cavity. If present in the pleural compartment, it indicates combined pneumothorax and pleural effusion. Rarely it may be seen in an obstructed oesophagus. It is a medical emergency if seen in the pulmonary trunk (air embolism). See differential diagnosis list (Appendix 3).

angel wing sign The lobes of the thymus are outlined by mediastinal air in neonates and young children with a pneumomediastinum.

anterior sulcus sign Also known as the 'double diaphragm sign'. It shows as a lucency over the upper quadrant when a pneumothorax is present in a supine patient. The free air lies in the anterior diaphragmatic sulcus, which is the uppermost portion of the thorax when the patient is supine. When detected, further views are required to establish the presence of the pneumothorax.

aortic nipple sign The left intercostal vein may drain anteriorly across the aortic arch to the innominate vein. This vein projects as a nipple on the aortic knuckle.

atelectasis Collapse and volume loss are synonymous terms.

atoll sign Cresentic regions of consolidation surround ground-glass opacity (resembling a coral atoll). A HRCT finding sometimes seen in COP.

B6 bronchus sign The B6 bronchus supplies the apical segment of the right lower lobe. When this segment is involved with consolidation or non-obstructing atelectasis, the B6 bronchus which passes anteroposteriorly is visible, projected just above the right hilum on the frontal view.

barrel chest Increased anteroposterior dimension seen in emphysema and indicating hyperinflation.

batwing distribution Colloquially called bat's wing shadowing. See Butterfly shadow.

beaded septum sign Small nodules may appear as a row of beads at a septum or fissure as an indication of lymphatic involvement. Lymphangitic carcinomatosis and sarcoidosis are the two main causes of this appearance.

big rib sign The ribs on the side of the patient closest to the X-ray tube (i.e. furthest from the film cassette) are magnified on the lateral CXR. This helps localisation of disease or a hemidiaphragm to the right or left side.

black bronchus sign The air within the bronchus is obviously blacker compared to the ground-glass opacity in the lungs. In normal lungs the blackness is only marginal.

black pleura sign The 'pleura' appears as a lucent line between the calcified pulmonary infiltrate (microlithiasis) and the adjacent ribs. In fact, the small subpleural cysts are outlined.

boot-shaped heart *Coeur en sabot* sign.

bronchial wall thickening Oedema, inflammatory cells or neoplastic cells infiltrate the peribronchial interstitial space. (See differential diagnosis of peribronchial cuffing, Appendix 3.)

bulging fissure sign If a consolidated lobe is swollen and enlarged, the fissure becomes displaced. The classic pneumonic process causing this is *Klebsiella* pneumonia (Friedlander bacillus); but it can also occur with *Haemophilus influenzae*, pneumococcal and tuberculous pneumonias.

butterfly (batwing) shadow This is the classic perihilar distribution of acute alveolar pulmonary oedema with a bilateral symmetric pattern. The central portion of the lungs shows shadowing (airspace filling) with the outer lung aerated. The reason/cause/mechanism may be due to the better lymphatic drainage in the outer portions of the lungs or the better aeration peripherally during the respiratory cycle.

calcification Deposition of calcium salts within a structure rendering it visible on X-ray examination. Includes dystrophic (degenerative) and metastatic (metabolic) calcification.

cavitation A cavity forms in an area of consolidation when necrosis occurs. Air enters the cavity when there is communication with the bronchial tree.

cervicothoracic sign This sign helps to indicate whether an upper mediastinal mass lies anteriorly or posteriorly. If a mass lies anteriorly, its upper border disappears as it approaches the clavicles. Because the posterior lung passes more highly, any posterior mediastinal mass outlined by the adjacent lung will show up above the clavicles.

***cœur en sabot* sign** The French *cœur en sabot* literally means the curved toe portion of a wooden shoe. It is the shape of the heart in tetralogy of Fallot where the apex points upwards and outwards due to the right ventricular hypertrophy.

comet tail sign On CT images, bronchovascular structures are twisted and coverge into the juxtapleural mass of 'rounded atelectasis' with the tail pointing towards the hilum. Also known as the talon sign, vacuum cleaner effect and helical effect. It has been likened to crow's feet and the cords of a parachute.

consolidation Filling of the airspaces with abnormal material such as transudate, exudate, cells or protein. Consolidated lung characteristically appears dense and shows the bronchi as air-filled tubular structures (see Air bronchogram sign) but obscures the underlying vessels.

continuous diaphragm sign The central junction between the two hemidiaphragms is normally not seen because of the heart. In cases of pneumomediastinum where gas is present extrapleurally between the heart and diaphragm, the central portion is also visualised. This sign can also be seen in the presence of a pneumopericardium.

corona radiata sign Numerous radiating strands ('spiculation') around the edge of a nodule which has a sunburst appearance. It usually indicates a bronchial carcinoma but rarely can be seen with infectious granulomas.

costal cartilage sign In men, the upper and lower portions of the costal cartilage become calcified first adjacent to the bony rib ends. In women, the central part of the costal cartilage adjacent to the rib calcifies first.

costal hook sign Segmental rib fractures will rotate into this configuration. This rotation is only possible if there is a further fracture within the same rib. It indicates a flail segment injury.

crow's feet sign Coarse bands of fibrosis (parenchymal bands) radiate from a thickened visceral pleural focus into the lungs. They may precede the development of rounded atelectasis in patients with asbestos exposure.

CT angiogram sign Pulmonary vessels are visualised on contrast-enhanced CT scanning against a background of relatively low attenuation material. It is seen with pneumonia, alveolar pulmonary oedema, alveolar cell carcinoma and lymphoma.

D sign A loculated pleural effusion will give a homogeneous peripheral opacity in the shape of a 'D'. When projected over the thoracic spine on the lateral CXR, it has been called the 'forward S' sign.

deep sulcus sign Pleural air collections in the supine patient lie anteriorly because this is the uppermost portion of the supine chest. The collected air makes the lateral costophrenic angle look deeper and the hemidiaphragm appears less dense. The signs of an apical pneumothorax, as would be seen on an erect CXR, are not present.

diaphragm flattening The height of the diaphragm apex is less than 1.5 cm to the line drawn between the costophrenic and the cardiophrenic sulci on the frontal film or between the anterior and posterior sulci on the lateral film.

double bronchial wall sign The bronchial wall is depicted occasionally in pneumomediastinum when air lies next to a central bronchus.

double contour sign The right heart border (right lateral margin of the right atrium) is normally outlined by the medial segment of the middle lobe. When the left atrium is enlarged, it bulges posteriorly and then at its side. The double contour is either the right margin of the left atrium lying densely behind the right heart border or, when massively dilated, extending beyond the right atrium.

double diaphragm sign There can be an impression of two hemidiaphragms in a supine patient with a pneumothorax. One outline is from the anterior pneumothorax air and the other is from the usual interface at the diaphragm apex. These may be visualised simultaneously. See anterior sulcus sign and deep sulcus sign.

eggshell calcification Hilar lymph nodes which have peripheral ring of calcification. Classically occurs with silicosis (5%) but can be mimicked by sarcoidosis, healed tuberculosis and treated lymphoma.

epicardial fat pad sign On the lateral CXR the normal pericardium is seen as a radiopaque line (less than 2 mm in thickness) between the anterior epicardial fat and the retrosternal pericardial fat. If the pericardium is thicker than 2 mm, pericardial thickening or an effusion is present.

extrapleural sign Expanding lesion in the parietal pleura or chest wall displacing the lung.

fallen lung sign This rare sign can occur if there is a bronchial fracture but the vascular pedicle remains intact. There is a pneumothorax and the lung sags downwards on an erect film and not inwards towards the hilum.

feeding vessel sign A distinct vessel leading to the apex of a peripheral area of consolidation.

figure 3 sign With aortic coarctation, the pre-stenotic and post-stenotic widening of the aorta may produce a 'figure 3' sign at the left border of the superior mediastinum.

flat waist sign The contours of the aortic knuckle and pulmonary artery become flattened in complete collapse of the left lower lobe due to leftward displacement and rotation of the heart.

Fleischner sign The hilum appears plump when there is a bulky embolus obstructing the main pulmonary artery at the hilum. This is highlighted by the decreased pulmonary artery branches beyond it.

floating hilum sign The 'clear space' between hilar lymphadenopathy and the mediastinum distinguishes it from mediastinal lymphadenopathy.

gloved finger shadow sign When bronchi become ectatic and filled with mucus, their tubular appearances resemble gloved fingers. One type is the 'toothpaste shadow' in allergic bronchopulmonary aspergillosis, where a band opacity of mucoid impaction points to the hilum.

Golden S sign See S sign of Golden.

ground-glass opacity This term describes a hazy increase in lung density. It must be subtle and not dense enough to obscure visualisation of the pulmonary vessels. It can be caused by air-space disease, interstitial thickening and even deflation.

halo sign A dense focal area of consolidation is surrounded by a halo of ground-glass opacity on CT scanning. It can be seen with haemorrhagic nodules such as Kaposi sarcoma and Wegener granulomatosis; and also seen in early invasive pulmonary aspergillosis.

Hampton hump sign A pulmonary infarct appears as a homogeneous wedge-shaped opacity with its base against the visceral pleura and a rounded apex directed towards the hilum. See Melting ice cube sign.

hanging drop heart The heart may appear normal in size, even though it is compromised, in chronic obstructive pulmonary disease by the hyperinflation of the lungs and depression of the hemidiaphragms.

head-cheese sign A mixture of lung attenuation with geographic areas of normal lung, ground-glass opacity and mosaic perfusion are seen on high-resolution CT. It resembles a sausage made from the head of a hog. It usually indicates infiltrative and obstructive disease. The common causes are sarcoidosis, hypersensitivity pneumonitis and infective bronchiolitis.

hilar convergence sign The convergence of the pulmonary arteries at the hilum is used to distinguish between a prominent hilum and an enlarged pulmonary artery.

hilum overlay sign If a structure is projected over the hilum, yet is separated from it, the hilar shape remains visible because of the adjacent aerated lung. This is different when a mass involves the hilum and the normal hilar configuration and outline are lost.

Hoffman–Rigler sign This is a superseded and complicated sign which indicates left ventricular enlargement on the lateral view by comparing the posterior border of the left ventricle to the inferior vena cava position.

honeycomb shadowing Cystic airspaces are apparent as ring shadows between coarse reticular shadowing. It implies destruction and fibrosis of alveolar walls and causes traction bronchiectasis.

hyperlucent hemithorax sign This sign can be due to a number of factors and occurs when there is unilateral hyperlucency or increased 'blackness'. It could be due to rotation, mastectomy, pneumothorax, previous surgery or reduced pulmonary vessels.

iceberg sign The top of thoraco-abdominal masses may be visible where they are in contact with the aerated lower lobes; but the lack of a lower border suggests that most of the mass lies in the abdomen. This sign can be seen in thoraco-abdominal aneurysms, oesophagogastric tumours, azygos continuations of the inferior vena cava and also retroperitoneal tumours extending into the thorax.

incomplete border sign This indicates that a CXR opacity is extraparenchymal, e.g. focal pleural disease. The inner border of the pleurally-based opacity is sharply defined but its outer margin fades off at an obtuse angle into the chest wall.

interface sign Nodular irregularity of bronchoarterial bundles in association with the beaded septum sign. Occurs in lymphangitis, carcinomatosis and sarcoidosis. Also used in CT to distinguish pleural fluid or ascites near the liver and spleen. With ascites the interface is sharp whereas with pleural fluid it is hazy.

juxtaphrenic peak sign In right upper lobe collapse, a small triangular shadow may obscure the dome of the right hemidiaphragm.

Kerley lines First described in 1933 by radiologist Dr Peter Kerley, who thought that they were due to engorged lymphatics. In 1951 he categorised the three patterns into A, B and C lines. These are septal lines that are thickened by fluid accumulation, cellular infiltration or connective tissue proliferation within the interlobular septa. They can be acute and transient, or chronic, due to lymphatic obstruction or fibrosis.

Kerley A lines are straight 2–6 cm lines, 1 mm in thickness, located in a radiating fashion midway between the hilum and pleura. They appear to cross over the bronchoarterial bundles.

Kerley B lines are 1 cm long, perpendicular to the lateral pleural surface. They are usually seen just above the costophrenic angles.

Kerley C lines are a fine network of superimposed Kerley B lines seen 'en face'.

Kreel's D lines are seen on the lateral CXR.

lemon sign Loculated effusion in the horizontal fissure which has the shape of a lemon including the small extensions at the margins.

luftsichel sign Occurs with left upper lobe collapse and is the paramediastinal translucency projected above the left hilum. It is derived from the German words *'Luft'* (air) and *'Sichel'* (sickle). The lucency is the aerated apex of the lower lobe positioned between the mediastinum and the collapsed left upper lobe. Originally it was thought to be due to herniation of the right lung across the midline. It needs to be distinguished from a loculated medial pneumothorax.

mass A discrete opacity greater than 3 cm in size.

melting ice cube sign A resolving pulmonary infarct maintains its homogeneity and wedge shape, unlike pneumonia, which resolves in a patchy manner.

meniscus sign A curved upper margin of a peripheral homogeneous opacity suggests a pleural effusion. It is due to the tapering split between the visceral and parietal pleural layers.

miliary pattern A collection of tiny discrete pulmonary opacities that are generally uniform in size (2 mm or less) and widespread in distribution.

mosaic pattern Regional differences in lung density are seen when there are areas of ground-glass opacity and areas of hypodense lung. The three basic causes are infiltrative lung disease, small airways disease and occlusive vascular disease. Constrictive obliterative bronchiolitis and multiple pulmonary emboli will produce hypodense lung with the blood shunted into the 'normal' ground-glass lung. These two processes can be distinguished by expiratory scans. Similar terms are mosaic perfusion and mosaic oligaemia.

mucoid impaction The presence of thick tenacious mucus within an airway produces band Y- or V-shaped opacities.

nodule A nodule is a mass less than 3 cm in size but the term can also be used interchangeably with mass. A nodular pattern is produced when rounded lesions accumulate in the interstitium.

Nordenstrom sign Lingular atelectasis which is associated with left lower lobe collapse.

oar rib The shape of the ribs in Mucopolysaccharidosis 1 (Hurler syndrome).

oesophageal tube displacement sign The oesophagus and oesophageal tube are displaced by haematoma when there is an aortic tear following trauma. Emergency aortography is indicated.

paratracheal stripe sign On a PA CXR, the right paratracheal stripe should be thin and becomes thickened with adjacent lymphadenopathy or haemorrhage. On the lateral CXR, the posterior margin of the trachea should be thin and, if it is thickened, adjacent pathology should be suspected.

pleural coif sign If a chest wall lesion has a detectable layer of extrapleural fat on its inner aspect, it can be localised unequivocally to the chest wall.

pleural tail sign A line shadow connecting a peripheral nodule to the pleura. Also known as a pleuropulmonary tail. This sign is not specific and is seen with a variety of lesions, both malignant and benign, particularly granulomas.

pneumorachis Air in the spinal canal. A rare sign as a result of trauma.

pruning of pulmonary arteries Rapid tapering from the enlarged central arteries to the peripheral arteries as seen in emphysema.

reticular shadowing Fine, medium or coarse irregular linear opacities due to interstitial thickening. When combined with nodular opacities it is described as a reticulonodular pattern.

reverse batwing sign With peripheral consolidation in chronic eosinophilic pneumonia, the perihilar lungs are clear.

reversed halo sign See atoll sign.

ring around the artery sign A well-defined lucent ring is seen around the right pulmonary artery on the lateral film in the presence of a pneumomediastinum.

S sign of Golden A right paramediastinal opacity with a margin of a reversed S is seen with a hilar malignant tumour obstructing the right upper lobe bronchus, causing collapse. The affected fissure has a central convexity because of the mass itself and a distal concave shape as a result of the collapse.

sabre sheath trachea sign The intrathoracic trachea shape can change in chronic obstructive pulmonary disease and can have a narrowed coronal width. Also called a scabbard trachea.

sail sign In neonates and young children, the shadow of the normal thymus is seen projecting laterally beyond the rest of the mediastinum. It must not be confused with a consolidated right upper lobe. See also the wave sign.

scimitar sign A curved band resembling a Turkish scimitar is the shadow produced by an anomalous pulmonary vein coursing through the lung and draining into a subdiaphragmatic inferior vena cava.

sentinel lines sign These lines can occur at the lung bases and be a sign of adjacent lower lobe volume loss. It is thought that they are due to bronchial kinking with distal atelectasis. They must be distinguished from other causes of plate-like atelectasis and septal lines. See Nordenstrom sign.

shaggy heart sign The pulmonary and pleural changes in asbestosis may partially blur the cardiac outline. Also seen with patchy consolidation adjacent to the heart as in pertussis pneumonia.

shifting granuloma sign If the position of a nodule shifts between examinations, it implies loss of volume in one part of the lung: an internal marker of atelectasis.

shrinking lungs Diaphragm dysfunction can occur in systemic lupus erythematous. The lungs lose volume as the diaphragm rises.

signet ring sign This is a sign of bronchiectasis and is seen when the segmental bronchus is larger in diameter than the accompanying pulmonary artery.

silhouette sign More accurately this should be called the 'loss of silhouette sign'. Whenever there is loss of a mediastinal border or diaphragmatic outline, it indicates that aerated lung is no longer outlining it. For instance, if there is loss of outline of the aortic knob it implies that there is a lesion or consolidation in the apicoposterior segment of the left upper lobe adjacent to the aortic knob.

snowman sign An unusual cardiac configuration due to total anomalous pulmonary venous drainage. The bottom of the snowman is the enlargement of the right atrium and ventricle. The top of the snowman is the superior mediastinal enlargement caused by the total anomalous pulmonary vein drainage into the superior vena cava or azygos vein. Other terms used to describe the cardiac shape are 'cottage loaf' or 'figure of 8'. The left side of the snowman's head is formed by the vertical vein (left anterior cardinal vein) draining all of the left pulmonary veins to the left brachiocephalic vein.

spinnaker sign Loculated air in a pneumomediastinum pushes the thymus into the shape of a spinnaker.

splaying of the carina sign Usually due to left atrial enlargement. Also known as the 'wishbone' sign.

split pleura sign Normally the opposed parietal and visceral pleura are not separated. Loculated fluid can, however, separate or split the thickened pleural envelope. The loculated fluid is usually lenticular in shape and infected. The subpleural fat adjacent to the parietal fluid can be thickened and oedematous. This sign can be useful in differentiating an empyema from a lung abscess. It can also be seen with haemothorax and talc pleurodesis.

third mogul sign Sometimes called the fourth mogul sign and is any abnormal protuberance of the left heart border on the frontal view. It could be due to an adjacent lesion or an enlarged left atrial appendage. A large left atrial appendage indicates mitral valve disease, i.e. 'mitralisation of the left heart border'. The first mogul is the aortic knob; the second mogul is the left main pulmonary artery; the other mogul is the cardiac apex.

thorn sign Shape of the fluid at the edge of a fissure adjacent to a pleural effusion.

thymic wave sign Impressions from the costochondral junctions may be seen on the normal thymic outline on the frontal film. This sign is not seen in thymic tumours or other anterior mediastinal masses.

toothpaste shadow Band shadow due to mucoid impaction with obstruction and distension of a bronchus (bronchocele). The distal lung remains aerated by collateral air drift.

tramline sign Parallel lines from ectatic bronchi which may also be thickened from chronic infections.

tree-in-bud sign Peripheral small centrilobular nodules are connected to linear branching opacities (terminal bronchioles) that resemble a tree in bud. This pattern is seen on thin-section CT but is not visible on chest radiographs. With endobronchial spread of disease, the terminal bronchioles become dilated and impacted with mucus and pus. It is most commonly seen in atypical *Mycobacterium* infection (NTM).

tubular artery sign Vessels may be outlined by air in a pneumomediastinum. Similar to 'ring around the artery' sign.

twiddling sign Rotation of the pacemaker device in the subcutaneous tissue of the chest wall with retraction of the leads. Presumably the device has been 'twiddled' by the patient.

upper triangle sign A triangular shadow is seen on the frontal radiograph resembling right upper lobe collapse when, in fact, there is collapse of the right lower lobe. It is caused by the rightward displacement of the upper mediastinum.

vanishing heart sign The margins of the heart become obscured in massive alveolar microlithiasis.

V sign of Naclerio Air along the diaphragm (horizontal) and para-oesophageal air (vertical) forms a 'V' and is an occasional sign on the frontal CXR in oesophageal tear.

vertebral fade-off sign There is decreasing density posteriorly on the lateral radiograph from the upper thoracic spine to the very lowest thoracic spine at the diaphragm. The vertebral fade-off sign occurs with increased density due to overlying lung disease (e.g. lower lobe collapse).

wandering wires Displacement of sternal cerlage wires following dehiscence of a median sternotomy.

water-bottle heart The heart shadow has a globular shape with a pericardial effusion or cardiomyopathy. Ebstein anomaly may have a similar shape.

waterfall sign Upper lobe fibrosis will elevate the hila. This causes the infrahilar pulmonary vessels to course downward more vertically than normal.

waterlily sign Hydatid cyst membranes floating on an air–fluid level indicate that the cyst has ruptured into a bronchus. Also known as the camelot sign.

wave sign The right thymic edge in young children has a wavy contour because it is indented by the anterior ribs. Also known as the notch sign.

Westermark sign There is relative lucency of a portion of lung distal to a large vessel embolus due to local oligaemia. This may be associated with enlargement of the ipsilateral main pulmonary artery (Fleischner sign). This sign can also occur with neoplastic destruction of a central pulmonary artery.

wishbone sign Splaying of the carina, usually due to left atrial enlargement.

APPENDIX 3

LISTS OF CAUSES AND DIFFERENTIAL DIAGNOSES

CAUSES OF SYMPTOMS

Chest pain

- Myocardial infarction
- Aortic dissection
- Pneumothorax
- Rib fractures
- Pneumonia
- Oesophageal rupture
- Pulmonary embolus

Dyspnoea

- Pulmonary embolus
- Emphysema
- Interstitial fibrosis
- Pneumothorax, pleural effusion
- Tracheal compression
- Anaemia
- Pulmonary oedema
- Asthma
- Diaphragm palsy
- Airway foreign body

Haemoptysis

- Pulmonary embolus
- Goodpasture syndrome
- Bronchiectasis
- Lung carcinoma
- Tuberculosis
- Coagulopathy
- Bronchitis
- Foreign body
- Catamenial
- MS

Pseudo-haemoptysis

- Upper GI bleeding
- Epistaxis
- Gingival or oral bleeding
- HHT

Cough

- Pneumonia
- Lung carcinoma
- Tracheal compression
- Chronic bronchitis
- Bronchiectasis
- Gastro-oesophageal reflux
- Goitre

Normal CXR and dyspnoea

- Pulmonary embolism

Women in labour with dyspnoea and shock

- Acute cardiogenic oedema
- Amniotic fluid embolism
- Massive gastric aspiration

Wheezing

- Asthma
- Foreign body
- Pulmonary oedema
- Pulmonary eosinophilia

DIFFERENTIAL DIAGNOSIS

MEDIASTINUM

Anterior mediastinal masses (5 T's)

- Thyroid
- Thymus
- Teratoma
- Terrible lymphoma
- Tortuous vessel

Middle mediastinal masses

- Aortic arch aneurysm
- Bronchogenic cyst
- Hiatal hernia
- Lymphadenopathy

Posterior mediastinal masses

- Neurogenic tumour
- Aneurysm of descending aorta
- Paraspinal lesion
- Extramedullary haemopoeisis
- Haematoma
- Lateral meningocoele

Shift of mediastinum to side of pathology

- Collapsed lung segments/lobe
- Surgical removal of lung segments/lobe
- Hypoplasia of lung segments/lobe

Mediastinal shift to side opposite pathology

- Large pleural mass or effusion
- Tension pneumothorax
- Foreign body (endobronchial—'ball valve')
- Bullae
- Diaphragmatic rupture/herniation

Pneumo-mediastinum in childhood

- Airway foreign body
- Asthma
- Pharyngeal perforation
- Oesophageal perforation
- Membranous croup

Pneumomediastinum

Spontaneous alveolar

- Rupture
- Asthma
- Croup
- Strenuous exercise
- Marijuana smoking
- Childbirth
- Vomiting
- Valsalva manoeuvre

Traumatic laceration

- Trachea
- Bronchus
- Lung
- Paranasal sinus (rare)

Perforation

- Pharynx
- Oesophagus (Boerhaave syndrome)

Extension

- Neck gas
- Retroperitoneal gas

Iatrogenic

- Recent thoracotomy
- Mediastinoscopy
- Over ventilation with PEEP
- Dental extraction (rare)

Pneumomediastinum mimics

- Pneumopericardium
- Medial pneumothorax
- Helium balloon of IACPB
- Mach band effect

SVC syndrome

- SVC obstruction
- Lymphoma
- Lymphadenopapthy

- Bronchogenic carcinoma (direct extension)
- Mediastinal fibrosis
- Irradiation
- Aortic aneurysm
- Goitre
- Pericardial effusion

Mediastinal lymphadenopathy

- Sarcoid
- Metastases
- Lymphoma
- TB and histoplasmosis

CARDIAC

Pulmonary arterial hypertension

Precapillary

- Chronic thromboemboli
- Chronic lung disease:
  - Emphysema
  - Chronic bronchitis
  - Interstitial fibrosis
  - Pleural fibrothorax
- Pulmonary vasculitis
- Eisenmenger syndrome
- Primary pulmonary hypertension

Over-circulation

- Atrial septal defect (ASD)
- Patent ductus arteriosus (PDA)
- Ventricular septal defect (VSD)

Postcapillary

- Left ventricular failure
- Mitral valve disease

Hypo-ventilation

- Obesity
- Sleep apnoea
- High altitude
- Chest wall deformity

Persistent left SVC

- Anatomical variant
- Heterotaxy syndromes
- Supracardiac TAPVR
- 'Vertical vein' of PAPVR
- Raghib syndrome (rare)

Enlarged central pulmonary arteries

- Pulmonary hypertension
- Post-stenotic dilatation
- Aneurysm

Left-to-right shunts

- ASD
- VSD
- PDA
- Gerbode defect
- PAPVR

Right-to-left shunts

- Tetralogy of Fallot
- Transposition of great vessels
- Eisenmenger syndrome

Prominent ascending ± arch

- Aneurysm
- Aortic valve disease
- Atherosclerosis
- Coarctation
- Pseudocoarctation
- Homocystinuria
- Marfan syndrome
- PDA
- Syphilitic aortitis
- Takayasu arteritis
- Tetralogy of Fallot

Gross cardiac enlargement

- Pericardial effusion
- Cardiomyopathy
- Valvular heart disease
- Ebstein anomaly

Small heart

- Emphysema (hanging drop heart)
- Addison disease
- Dehydration
- Constrictive pericarditis
- Malnutrition
- Senile atrophy

Upper lobe blood diversion

- Rise in pulmonary venous pressure
- Lower zone disease e.g. IPF, emphysema
- PE occlusions in lower zones

Large cardiac silhouette and normal pulmonary vascularity

- Pericardial effusion
- Ebstein anomaly
- Treated left ventricular failure

DIAPHRAGM

Elevated hemidiaphragm

- Normal variant (eventration, diaphragm thinning)
- Splinting of diaphragm (acute abdominal or thoracic conditions)
- Elevation, secondary to lobar collapse
- Subpulmonary effusion
- Phrenic nerve paralysis
- Raised intra-abdominal pressure
- Diaphragmatic rupture/ herniation
- Hemiplegia
- Gaseous distension of stomach (left)

Small lungs

- Expiration
- Interstitial fibrosis
- Bilateral lobar collapse
- Bilateral elevated diaphragms
- Obesity
- Ascites
- Term pregnancy

HILA

Hilar lymphadenopathy

- Sarcoid
- Metastases
- Lymphoma
- Primary tuberculosis (TB)
- 'Reactive' to infection
- DD large pulmonary arteries

Unilateral hilar enlargement

- Central bronchogenic carcinoma
- Metastatic lymphadenopathy
- Lymphoma
- Inflammatory lymphadenopathy
- Pulmonary embolism (Fleischner sign)
- Blocked contralateral pulmonary artery

Hilar eggshell calcification

- Silicosis
- Sarcoidosis
- Lymphoma following radiotherapy
- Embolism
- Chronic embolism

Aorto-pulmonary window/left suprahilar mass

- Bronchogenic carcinoma
- Bulky lymphadenopathy
- Bronchogenic cyst
- Thymic neoplasm
- Aneurysm/vascular ectasia

PLEURA

Pleural calcification

- Previous pleural TB
- Previous empyema
- Previous haemothorax
- Asbestos plaques

Pleural effusion

- Transudate (protein <3 g/dL):
  - Cardiac failure
  - Hypoalbuminaemia

  - Renal failure
  - Meigs syndrome
  - Peritoneal dialysis
- Exudate (protein > 3g/dL):
  - Infection
  - Malignancy
  - Pulmonary embolus
  - Collagen diseases
  - Subphrenic abscess
  - Pancreatitis
  - Asbestos
- Haemorrhagic:
  - Trauma
  - Thoracotomy
  - Pulmonary infarct
- Chylous:
  - Obstructed thoracic duct
  - Lymphangioleiomyomatosis (LAM)

Combined pleural and pericardial effusions

- SLE
- Infection (TB, viral)
- Tumour (metastases, lymphoma)
- Churg–Strauss syndrome
- Myxoedema
- Dressler syndrome

Pleural mass mimics

- Loculated effusion
- Haematomas
- Pleural plaque
- Lymphoma of chest wall
- Peripheral lung lesion

Acute abdominal disease with pleural effusions

- Pancreatitis
- Subphrenic abscess
- Perinephric abscess
- Trauma
- Leaking aneurysm
- Incarcerated diaphragmatic hernia
- Amoebic abscess

Pneumothorax

- Spontaneous:
  - Apical blebs
  - Chronic obstructive pulmonary disease
  - Asthma
  - Cavitating pneumonia
  - Cystic fibrosis
  - Interstitial fibrosis
  - Pleural metastases
  - Pulmonary Langerhans cell histiocytosis (PLCH)
  - LAM/tuberous sclerosus
  - Catamenial pneumothorax
  - Connective tissue disorders
  - Pneumomediastinum extension
  - Pneumoperitoneum extension
  - Bronchopleural fistula
- Traumatic:
  - Blunt or penetrating injury
  - Thoracotomy
  - Pleural aspiration
  - Percutaneous lung biopsy
  - Transbronchial lung biopsy
  - Central venous line insertion
  - Barotrauma

LUNGS

Unilateral 'white-out'

- Massive pleural effusion
- Previous pneumonectomy
- Lung atelectasis
- Lung aplasia or agenesis
- Pleural mesothelioma
- Complete TB fibrothorax

Increased density of a hemithorax

- Consolidation
- Pleural effusion
- Collapse
- Carcinoma, mesothelioma
- Post-pneumonectomy
- Fibrothorax
- Haemorrhage

Multiple pulmonary calcifications

- Infection:
  - TB (not miliary)
  - Histoplasmosis, coccidioidomycosis
  - Chicken pox
- Metastases
- Mitral valve disease
- Alveolar microlithiasis
- Hyperparathyroidism

Ground glass on CXR

- Acute symptoms:
  - Oedema
  - Haemorrhage
  - Infection
  - Acute interstitial pneumonia
- Chronic symptoms:
  - Hypersensitivity pneumonia
  - Usual interstitial pneumonia
  - Non-specific interstitial pneumonia
  - Desquamative interstitial pneumonia/respiratory bronchiolitis (RB-ILD)
  - Alveolar proteinosis (PAP)

Types of pulmonary collapse

- Obstructive
- Passive atelectasis
- Adhesive atelectasis
- Cicatrising atelectasis

Collapse (lung, lobar, segmental)

- Mucus plug (postoperative, asthma)
- Bronchogenic neoplasm
- Foreign body
- Endotracheal tube down bronchus
- Extrinsic lymph node compression
- Stricture:
  - Post-inflammatory
  - Post-radiotherapy

Alveolar filling consolidation

- Acute—infection, haemorrhage, oedema
- Chronic—alveolar cell carcinoma, alveolar proteinosis

Lobar pneumonia

- Streptococcuspneumoniae (commonest)
- Klebsiella pneumoniae (bulging fissures)
- Staphylococcus aureus
- TB

Peripheral lung consolidation

- Bacterial pneumonia
- COP
- Chronic eosinophilic pneumonia
- Pulmonary infarction
- MALT lymphoma
- Sequestrated lung

Antibiotic-resistant cavitary pneumonia

- TB
- Atypical mycobacteria
- Nocardia
- Fungal pneumonia
- Sequestrated lung

Non-thrombotic pulmonary emboli

- Septic emboli
- Catheter embolism
- Fat embolism
- Venous air embolism
- Amniotic fluid embolism
- Tumour embolism
- Talc embolism
- Vertebroplasty cement
- Rare: iodinated oil, mercury, cotton, hydatid, trophoblastic embolism

Septic pulmonary emboli

- Tricuspid valve endocarditis
- Infected catheters and pacemaker wires
- Peripheral septic thrombophlebitis
- Intravenous drug abuse
- Organ transplants

Calcified pulmonary emboli

- Chronic thrombo-embolism (rarely)
- Calcifying atrial myoma

- Bone fragment (bone marrow transplant)
- Calcified tumour-thrombus (metastatic renal carcinoma)
- Villotrophoblastic pulmonary emboli
- Vertebroplasty cement

Fat embolism syndrome

- Trauma
- Haemoglobinopathy (sickle cell disease)
- Severe burns
- Soft tissue injuries
- Diabetes mellitus
- Pancreatitis
- Severe infection
- Neoplasms
- Osteomyelitis
- Blood transfusion
- Cardiopulmonary bypass
- Altitude decompression
- Suction lipectomy
- Renal transplantation
- Alcoholism
- Inhalational anaesthesia

Lucent lung fields

- Technique
- COPD
- Asthma
- Air trapping with foreign body
- Pulmonary oligogaemia

Decreased pulmonary flow

- Cardiac tamponade
- Constrictive pericarditis
- Fibrosing mediastinitis
- Right to left shunt
- Addison disease

Unilateral hypertranslucency

- Chest wall:
  - Mastectomy
  - Scoliosis
  - Polio
  - Poland syndrome (unilateral absent pectoral muscle)

- Pulmonary:
  - Unilateral bullae
  - Compensatory hyperinflation
  - Swyer–James/MacLeod syndrome
  - Unilateral major embolus
  - Congenital lobar emphysema
  - Obstructive hyperaeration
- Pleura:
  - Pneumothorax
  - Contralateral pleural effusion (supine film)
  - Rotation

Cystic lung disease

- Emphysema
- Cystic bronchiectasis
- LAM/tuberous sclerosis
- Cystic metastases
- Wegener granulomatosis
- PCP
- Septic pulmonary emboli
- Interstitial fibrosis (honeycombing)
- Papillomatosis

Increased interstitial markings

- Interstitial pulmonary oedema
- Acute interstitial pneumonia
- Chronic bronchitis
- Lymphangitis carcinomatosa
- PCP
- Sarcoidosis
- Interstitial fibrosis (drugs, connective tissue disease, asbestosis, idiopathic)

Interstitial idiopathic (most fibrosis common cause)

- Collagen disease (rheumatoid, scleroderma, systemic lupus erythematosus [SLE])
- Asbestosis, silicosis
- Drugs (amiodarone, nitrofurantoin, cytotoxics, methysergide)
- Paraquat poisoning

Bronchiectasis

- Post-infectious:
  - TB, bacterial or viral pneumonia
  - Recurrent sinus infection
- Congenital:
  - Dyskinetic ciliary syndrome
  - Kartagener syndrome
  - Williams–Campbell syndrome
  - Mounier–Kuhn syndrome
  - Sequestrated lung
  - Cystic fibrosis
- Obstruction:
  - Cancer
  - TB stenosis
  - Inhaled foreign body
- Bronchopulmonary aspergillosis
- Hypogammaglobulinaemia
- Chronic aspiration
- Traction (interstitial fibrosis)

Central bronchiectasis

- ABPA
- Cystic fibrosis
- TB
- Mounier–Kuhn syndrome
- Williams–Campbell syndrome
- Radiation fibrosis

Upper lobe fibrosis

- TB, histoplasmosis
- Sarcoid
- Extrinsic allergic alveolitis (chronic)
- Radiation
- Progressive massive fibrosis
- Ankylosing spondylitis

Apical cap

- Non-granulomatous scarring
- Granulomatous scarring
- Post-irradiation fibrosis
- Pancoast tumour
- Extrapleural haematoma
- Extrapleural fat

CXR air-fluid levels

- Lung cavities (see below)
- Hydropneumothorax
- Haemopneumopericardium
- Dilated oesophagus
- Hiatal hernia
- Haemopneumothorax:
  - Spontaneous pneumothorax with bleeding
  - Iatrogenic
  - Trauma
- Chest wall abscess

Diffuse alveolar haemorrhage

- Bleeding disorders
- Any cause of haemoptysis and complicated by aspiration
- Goodpasture syndrome
- SLE
- Wegener granulomatosis
- Systemic vasculitis
- Drugs
- Blunt chest trauma
- Idiopathic pulmonary haemosiderosis

Pulmonary infiltrates with eosinophilia (pulmonary eosinophilia ± blood eosinophilia)

- Leoffler syndrome (simple eosinophilic pneumonia)
- Chronic eosinophilic pneumonia
- Acute eosinophilic pneumonia
- Idiopathic hypereosinophilic syndrome (eosinophilic leukaemia)
- Churg–Strauss syndrome

Migratory lung opacities (fleeting shadows)

- Organising pneumonia
- Eosinophilic lung disease
- Pulmonary alveolar proteinosis
- Diffuse alveolar haemorrhage
- Recurrent aspiration
- Wegener granulomatosis
- Churg–Strauss syndrome

Granulomatous disease

- TB
- MAC
- Sarcoid
- Wegener granulomatosis
- Lymphomatoid granulomatosis
- Allergic granulomatosis (Churg–Strauss syndrome)
- Bronchocentric granulomatosis
- PLCH

Solitary pulmonary nodule (coin lesion)

- Tumours (bronchial cancer, metastasis, adenoma)
- Granuloma, usually tuberculoma
- Hamartoma
- Chest wall lesions:
  - Pleural mesothelioma
  - Pleural fibroma
  - Skin tumour
  - Nipple
- Others:
  - Rounded pneumonia
  - Rheumatoid nodule
  - Hydatid, haematoma
  - Arteriovenous fistula
  - Paraffinoma
  - Bronchial cyst

Cavitating lung lesion

- Infection—TB:
  - Hydatid
  - Pyogenic
  - Fungal
- Tumours:
  - Primary squamous
  - Secondary squamous
- Collagen diseases—rheumatoid
- Wegener disease
- Infarct
- Haematoma
- Progressive massive fibrosis
- Sequestrated segment
- Cystic bronchiectasis
- DD blebs, bullae, pneumatocoele

Intracavitary mass

- Necrotic carcinoma
- Haematoma
- Fungal ball
- Complicated hydatid cyst
- Rasmussen aneurysm

Miliary nodules

- Miliary tuberculosis
- Miliary metastases
- Sarcoidosis
- Silicosis
- Fungal diseases:
  - Histoplasmosis
  - Coccidioidodomycosis

Small nodular pattern (1–5 mm nodules)

- Metastases:
  - Thyroid, breast, renal
- Lymphoma
- Interstitial granulomas:
  - Sarcoidosis
  - Chronic hypersensitivity pneumonitis
  - PLCH
  - Miliary infections (TB, cryptococcus, coccidioidomycosis and histoplasmosis)
  - Wegener granulomatosis
  - Lymphomatoid granulomatosis
- Pneumoconiosis:
  - Silicosis, coal workers' pneumoconiosis, beryllosis and talcosis

Large nodules

- Metastases
- Abscesses
- Rheumatoid disease
- Wegener granulomatosis
- MALT lymphoma

Cannonball metastases

- Colonic carcinoma
- Testicular tumours

- Soft tissue sarcomas
- Sarcomatous

Multiple bilateral opacities

- Metastases
- Infection
- COP
- Chronic eosinophilic pneumonia
- Vasculitis
- PE

Rapidly progressive pulmonary nodules

- Fungal pneumonia
- Septic emboli
- Tuberculous infection
- Fulminant metastatic
- disease
- Haemorrhagic metastatic disease

Small lungs

- Expiration
- Interstitial fibrosis
- Bilateral lobar collapse
- Bilateral elevated diaphragms
- Obesity
- Ascites
- Term pregnancy

Endobronchial mass

- Carcinoma
- Carcinoid
- Metastatic deposit
- Mucous gland adenoma
- Leiomyoma
- (Foreign body)

Benign mimics of bronchogenic carcinoma

- Non-calcified granulomas
- Pneumonia
- Rounded atelectasis
- Progressive massive fibrosis
- Wegener granulomatosis
- Nipple shadow

PULMONARY OEDEMA

Pulmonary oedema

- Heart failure
- Renal failure
- Liver failure
- Aspiration
- Chest trauma
- Drug hypersensitivity
- Drug overdose (heroin)
- Fluid overload
- High altitude
- Inhalation of toxic agents
- Intracranial disease
- Near drowning
- Oxygen toxicity
- Shock lung
- Transfusion reaction

Acute pulmonary oedema with normal sized heart

- Myocardial infarct
- Acute cardiac arrhythmia
- Fluid overload
- 'Non-cardiogenic' pulmonary oedema

Unilateral pulmonary oedema

- Prolonged lateral decubitus position
- Unilateral aspiration
- Pulmonary contusion
- Thoracentesis
- Bronchial obstruction

Hydrostatic pulmonary oedema

- Volume overload
- Renal failure:
  - Over-hydration
- Decreased oncotic pressure:
  - Hypoalbuminaemia
- Heart disease—'cardiogenic':
  - Mitral stenosis/regurgitation
  - Acute myocardial infarction
  - Acute arrhythmia

- Left ventricular aneurysm
- Pulmonary veno-occlusive disease

Non-cardio-genic oedema without diffuse alveolar damage

- Drug reaction
- Drug overdose
- Transfusion reaction
- Neurogenic:
  - Head trauma
  - Seizures
  - Intracranial haemorrhage
  - Tumour
- High altitude
- Near drowning
- Aspiration
- Chest trauma

Peribronchial cuffing

- Asthma
- Chronic bronchitis
- Interstitial pulmonary oedema
- Viral pneumonia

Kerley B lines

- Congestive heart failure
- Lymphangitic carcinoma
- *Mycoplasma,* viral and *Pneumocystis carinii* pneumonia
- Interstitial fibrosis
- Sarcoid

Diffuse alveolar damage

- Idiopathic—acute interstitial pneumonia
- Risk factors:
  - Adult respiratory distress syndrome
  - Sepsis
  - Shock
  - Aspiration
  - Pneumonia
  - Trauma (direct lung trauma and fat embolism)
  - Pancreatitis
  - Radiation
  - Toxic gas inhalation

- Near drowning
- Drugs
- Transfusional reaction (TRALI)

BONES

Inferior rib notching

- Coarctation
- Tetralogy of Fallot (unilateral, usually left side)
- Blalock–Taussig shunt (unilateral right)
- Neurofibromatosis
- Vena caval obstruction
- Pulmonary atresia

Superior rib notching

- Quadriplegia
- Poliomyelitis
- Rheumatoid arthritis
- Scleroderma

GENERAL

Abnormal air collections

- Subcutaneous emphysema
- Pneumothorax
- Pneumomediastinum
- Pulmonary interstitial emphysema
- Lung cavity
- Air embolism

Dilated oesophagus

- Above an oesophageal stricture
- Achalasia
- Scleroderma
- Chagas disease

Smoking-induced lung disease

- Bronchogenic carcinoma
- Emphysema
- Chronic bronchitis
- CPFE
- Histiocytosis x (PLCH)
- Respiratory bronchiolitis (RB-ILD)
- DIP

Inthoracic lesions containing fat

- Hamartoma
- Diaphragmatic hernia
- Pleural lipoma
- Mediastinal lipomatosis
- Thymolipoma
- Germ cell tumours

HPOA

- Pulmonary:
  - Bronchogenic carcinoma (usually squamous)
  - TB
  - Abscesses
  - Bronchiectasis
  - Emphysema
  - PCP in AIDS
  - Hodgkin disease
  - Metastases
  - Cystic fibrosis
- Pleural:
  - Fibroma
- Abdominal:
  - Liver cirrhosis
  - Whipple disease
  - Gastric neoplasm
  - Pancreatic neoplasm
  - Bowel lymphoma
- Cardiac:
  - Cyanotic congenital heart disease

INDEX

References to figures and tables are in *italics*.

R